Psychobiology of
Language

MIT Press Studies in Neuropsychology and Neurolinguistics
David Caplan, series editor

Psychobiology of Language, edited by Michael Studdert-Kennedy, 1983

Psychobiology of Language

Edited by Michael Studdert-Kennedy

The MIT Press
Cambridge,
Massachusetts
London, England

The Work Session that provided a beginning for the development
of this book was held at the Neurosciences Research Program,
Jamaica Plain, Massachusetts, on March 22–24, 1981, under the
chairmanship of Harold Goodglass and Michael Studdert-Kennedy.
The collaborative authorship involving all participants proceeded
after this date under the editorial guidance of Michael Studdert-
Kennedy.

Second printing, 1984

This book was set in Times Roman
by The MIT Press Computergraphics Department

Library of Congress Cataloging in Publication Data

Main entry under title:

Psychobiology of language.
   (MIT Press studies in neuropsychology and neurolinguistics)
   Bibliography: p.
   Includes index.
   1. Neurolinguistics—Addresses, essays, lectures.
2. Language disorders—Addresses, essays, lectures.
3. Psychobiology—Addresses, essays, lectures.
I. Studdert-Kennedy, Michael. II. Series.
QP399.P79 1983   612'.78   83–972
ISBN 0–262–19217–9
ISBN 0-262-69310-0

Contents

Contents

PART V

PART VI

Series Foreword

The MIT Press Studies in Neuropsychology and Neurolinguistics present theoretical and empirical research on the neural mechanisms underlying language and cognition and their pathologies. These studies focus on two lines of investigation. The first is the application of concepts and methods of study of normal language and cognition to the investigation of their disturbances. The second is the use of increasingly detailed observational techniques in the clinical and basic neurosciences to deepen our understanding of the neural bases for language and cognition, normal and disturbed. The scope of the studies is broad and includes non-human species as well as man, developmental issues, and related areas. It is intended to make available significant new work in neuropsychology and neurolinguistics that requires book-length treatment, and its goal is to serve as a vehicle for the dissemination of new approaches, ideas, and results and as a catalyst for new research efforts.

The members of the advisory board for The MIT Press Studies in Neuropsychology and Neurolinguistics are

Maureen Dennis
The Hospital for Sick Children, Toronto

Steven Hilliard
University of California at San Diego

Patricia Goldman-Rakic
Yale University

Marc Jeannerod
INSERM, Lyon

Scott Kelso
Haskins Laboratories

Larry Squires
University of California at
San Diego

André Roch Lecours
University of Montreal

Edgar B. Zurif
City University of New York
and Brandeis University

John C. Marshall
Oxford University

David Caplan

Preface

This is the first Neurosciences Research Program publication on language since Eric Lenneberg's 1974 *Bulletin* entitled *Language and Brain: Developmental Aspects*. In the interim, much has happened to sharpen our view of how we might best approach the biology of language. In particular, the linguist's description of language as an autonomous cognitive system, comprising the autonomous subsystems of phonology and syntax, has penetrated neighboring fields and raised the question of the extent to which this description might validly be extended into psychology and neuropsychology. The importance of this question for our understanding of the biological status of language was deemed sufficient to make it the focus of an NRP Work Session.

The first five parts of the book follow the organization of the Work Session: an introduction, perceptuomotor, lexical, and syntactic processes, and prospects for future neuroanatomical studies by stimulation mapping and measures of cerebral metabolism. The sixth part of the book is a chapter of concluding comments. Within each of the first four parts at least one chapter treats the topic from a linguistic, psychological, or neuropsychological point of view; an exception is part II, for which Mark Liberman's chapter in part I may be read as offering a linguistic view. The parts themselves are revised and, in many cases, much expanded versions of the oral presentations made by the participants.

The comments that follow many of the chapters and that constitute part VI summarize and often elaborate on the original discussions. The editor prepared these comments from written summaries and tape recordings of the proceedings and from his own prejudices. With a few exceptions (where the remarks of a particular individual provided the main, or only, substantive points of discussion), the sources of the various arguments, comments, and criticisms are not indicated.

I am indebted to many people for their help and guidance. First, I thank Frederic Worden and Alvin Liberman for encouraging me to undertake the project, Harold Goodglass for his share in organizing it, and the staff of NRP for their hard work in carrying it through. Next, I thank Lise Menn and Robert Remez for their careful and substantial summaries of the Work Session's presentations and discussions, prepared from their notes and from tape recordings; without these summaries, my own work would have been vastly increased. Finally, I thank George Adelman for his patience with my dilatory habits and for his expert editorial advice.

Michael Studdert-Kennedy

Participants

Ursula Bellugi
The Salk Institute for
Biological Studies
La Jolla, CA

D. Frank Benson
Department of Neurology
University of California
Medical School
Los Angeles, CA

David Caplan
Division of Neurology
Ottawa Civic Hospital
Ottawa, Ontario

Maureen Dennis
Department of Psychology
The Hospital for Sick Children
Toronto, Ontario

John C. Fentress
Departments of Biology and
Psychology
Dalhousie University
Halifax, Nova Scotia

Lauren K. Gerbrandt
Neurosciences Research
Program
Jamaica Plain, MA

Norman Geschwind
Neurological Unit
Beth Israel Hospital
Boston, MA

Harold Goodglass
Psychology Service
Boston Veterans
Administration Medical
Center
Boston, MA

Alvin M. Liberman
Haskins Laboratories
New Haven, CT

Mark Y. Liberman
Bell Laboratories
Murray Hill, NJ

Lise Menn
Aphasia Research Center
Department of Neurology
Boston University School of
Medicine
Boston, MA

Lawrence J. Mononen*
Behavioral Sciences Group
Wang Laboratories
Lowell, MA

Morris Moscovitch
Department of Psychology
Erindale College
Mississauga, Ontario

George A. Ojemann
Department of Neurological
Surgery
University of Washington
School of Medicine
Seattle, WA

Zenon W. Pylyshyn
Department of Psychology
University of Western Ontario
London, Ontario

Robert E. Remez
Department of Psychology
Barnard College
New York, NY

Francis O. Schmitt
Neurosciences Research
Program
Jamaica Plain, MA

Michael Studdert-Kennedy
Queens College
City University of New York
Flushing, NY

Frederic G. Worden
Neurosciences Research
Program
Jamaica Plain, MA

Eran Zaidel
Department of Psychology
University of California at
Los Angeles
Los Angeles, CA

Edgar B. Zurif
Graduate Center
City University of New York
New York, NY
and Brandeis University
Waltham, MA

*NRP staff coordinator at the
time of the Work Session

PART I

What is language? Can we distinguish language from general cognition? Is language an isolable, biologically coherent system? Does the linguistic description of language as an autonomous system, formed from a combination of more or less autonomous subsystems, correspond to psychological and neurophysiological fact? These and related topics are the themes of the discussions that follow, and perhaps an initial word of justification is called for.

From a biological point of view we may raise the issue of the autonomy of language, simply because there can be no biology of language if language is not, in some sense, a separate system. Yet no behavioral system—indeed, no organ—can be entirely independent of other characteristics of an animal. The unit of natural selection is the individual, not the gene, or even the gene complex. Moreover, the unit is the individual in relation to other individuals—very obviously so in the case of interlocking patterns of social behavior, such as language.

As a simple instance of this lack of autonomy, consider the lexicon, constrained in content by individual and social cognitive demand, in form by perceptuomotor capacity. To categorize and differentiate among many thousands of objects, events, and attributes is not in itself linguistic, even if the capacity seems only to emerge through language. The impulse to name—in the child no less than in the adult, in the primitive society with its often vast inventories of flora and fauna (Lévi-Strauss, 1966) no less than in industrial society with its diverse technologies and subcultures—is logically prior to the instrument of naming, phonology. And phonology, however arbitrary, abstract and "unnatural" its particulars may often seem, is nonetheless grounded in and constrained by anatomy and physiology. The segmental structure of the lexicon, that is, the few dozen phonetic segments (consonants and vowels) from which, by permutation and combination, every language constructs its lexicon, is a solution—perhaps a biologically unique solution—to the problem of matching a finite set of articulators to the cognitive demand for a more or less unlimited lexicon.

Whether this segmental structure requires specialized systems of perception and motor control is of great interest and a question to which several of the following discussions are directly, or indirectly, addressed. But we can hardly doubt that phonological form reflects not only anatomical and physiological constraints on movement but also the perceptual modality to which the movements are addressed. This truth has been borne in on us in recent years by the discovery of American Sign Language (ASL). (Klima and Bellugi, 1979; and see the chapter by Bellugi). Briefly, we now know that ASL (and, without a doubt, British, Chinese, Russian, Brazilian, and many other sign languages) has evolved entirely independently, and yet with a dual structure exactly analogous to that of spoken language. Every meaningful sign is formed by some distinctive combination drawn from a few dozen hand configurations, hand orientations, places of articulation, and movements, each in itself meaningless; the signs are then modulated and ordered syntactically to form an utterance. What is of interest here is, first, that the overall formational structures of spoken and signed morphemes seem to be largely determined by their modalities of expression: a sequential pattern in time addressed to the ear or a layered pattern in space addressed to the eye (Studdert-

Kennedy and Lane, 1980). A second point is that the predominantly sequential structure of speech and the predominantly layered, parallel structure of ASL extend even into the syntactic structures of the two modes of language (Bellugi, 1980a); the syntactic sanctum is not inviolate. But this is not the place to elaborate these matters (see the chapter by Bellugi). Enough has been said to make it obvious that there are no grounds for expecting language to be free of its moorings in the perceptuomotor systems from which it has emerged. We do not talk with our toes.

In fact, we may even hope to gain some insight into the nature of language by exploring its perceptuomotor origins. Consider, for example, the notion of Lenneberg (1967) that the hierarchical, interdigitated, interlocking pattern of activity in synergistic groups of muscles marshaled for speaking is not only formally analogous to, but functionally continuous with, the hierarchical patterns of organization at phonemic, morphemic, and syntactic levels of description. Lenneberg (1967, p. 106) wrote that "formal aspects of purely physiological processes seem to be similar to certain formal aspects of grammatical processes . . . as if the two, physiology and syntax, were intimately related, one grading into the other. . . ." In other words, linguistic structure may emerge from, and may even be viewed as, a special case of motoric structure, the structure of action. This is a view with which Herbert Spencer, the first great evolutionary psychologist, would not have been uncomfortable.

A similar argument was elaborated by A. M. Liberman (1970), from a perceptual point of view, when he drew attention to formal similarities between the processes of decoding phonetic and syntactic structures. He described the analogies between the overlapping actions of separate muscles as they merge to form a syllable and the interleaving of deep structure segments to form the complex utterance. And he emphasized the need for a specialized decoding device for the comprehension of both phonological and syntactic structures.

An important point here is that despite the possible continuity between physiology and syntax, the true coherence of language may rest on a physiologically novel use of segmented structure, at two functionally distinct, yet hierarchically related, levels of organization: syntax and phonology. So far as we know such a dual structure—echoed, perhaps, in the structures of music and dance—is without biological parallel. Here, then, may be a sense in which language is indeed autonomous: not fully separable, but different, a subsystem (itself a nesting of subsystems) nested within the organism, and subject to idiosyncratic principles, just as are hearing and sight within the broad cross-modal structure of perception.

A Linguistic Approach   M. Y. Liberman

I shall attempt to sketch what linguistics can contribute to
a discussion of the biological autonomy of spoken language,
relying as little as possible on the details of one or another
school's theories, but staying as specific as the nature of the
occasion permits. I shall describe some aspects of spoken
language that are often argued to be "autonomous," in the
sense of that word as used by linguists, and suggest some of
the reasons that such arguments are plausible, concentrating
on some characteristics of spoken language that are perhaps
so commonplace as to be in danger of being ignored.

First, we must observe that linguists use the term "autonomy" primarily to mean formal separateness or distinc-
tiveness of descriptive apparatus, so that the claim that
"syntax is autonomous," for instance, is taken to mean that
the system of description appropriate for syntactic phenomena is based on a set of primitive elements and relations
different from those appropriate for other aspects of human
cognition, that syntactic regularities can be stated without
reference to entities outside this set (for example, those appropriate to phonology or to semantics), and so forth. It is
worth noting that such a concept of autonomy is logically
independent from issues of neurological autonomy; it is conceivable that linguistic systems could be autonomous in this
formal sense and still be implemented by circuitry that is of
a standard type or is shared by other faculties or scattered

among a number of areas. The overused analogy of the digital computer makes the logic of this point clear—formally autonomous software (for instance, a data-base management system or a speech synthesizer) may share identical hardware; and alternatively, the same program may use different physical devices on different occasions, as when different chunks of memory or disk storage are allocated to it by the operating system. It is likely that biological systems are somewhat less perverse in their separation of form and function, but we should still be wary of the naive expectation that autonomy in cognitive and behavioral systems will necessarily have precise anatomical correlates. Anatomy aside, however, I think it is generally reasonable to expect that cognitive or behavioral autonomy will generally be associated with some degree of biological specialization. Even if the system in question is initially just a special usage of a more general faculty, evolution can be expected to seize the opportunity to develop and adapt if the system increases individual fitness.

Let me begin by listing three characteristics that all known spoken languages share: (1) a large, indefinitely extensible set of words, whose articulatory/acoustic definition is mediated by a phonological system; (2) a syntactic system, that is, a set of normative principles governing the form and order of words combined into phrases, principles that cannot be explained by appeal to the nature of the concepts such phrases are used to express; (3) a propensity for constant change, which characteristically results in systematic differentiation by sex, class, location, and so forth.

Speakers seem to learn, or to invent, at least as many words as they need; often words seem to be multiplied beyond necessity, out of pedantry, as shibboleths, or for the simple fun of it. Seashore and Erickson (1940) estimated the recognition vocabulary of the average college student at 156,000 words, and using the same method, Smith (1941) estimated the recognition vocabulary of the average first grader at

24,000 words. As Miller (1951, p. 149) writes, "As a general rule, the estimated size of the vocabulary is proportional to the size of the dictionary used to supply the test words." Since the dictionary used in obtaining these estimates did not include slang, most proper names, or specially defined phrases (for example, "solar cell," which is not a dungeon with a south-facing window), the estimates could doubtless be increased. For highly educated people or for speakers of several languages estimates several times higher seem possible. Of course, individuals' active vocabularies are generally much smaller, with estimates of 5,000 to 10,000 words being reasonable (Miller, 1951, p. 121). Reliable estimates for recognition vocabularies of individuals in nonliterate cultures are not, as far as I know, available; in any case, my point here is simply that spoken languages are not stingy about vocabulary size. Cultures and subcultures add words freely, as circumstances dictate, with no apparent concern about exhausting a limited capacity. The existence of malapropisms shows that individuals' capacity to keep so many words distinct is sometimes overloaded, but most such errors are individual, sporadic, and a source of amusement to others. This combination of large set size and distinctness (both in principle and in practice) of individual set members requires a striking set of abilities in memory, motor control, and perception; like other striking species-specific capabilities, this one might be taken as prima facie evidence of specialization.

This wealth of words is somehow mapped into noises made by our eating and breathing apparatus.[1] The details of the mapping between words and sounds suggest an intermediate representation, usually called "phonological." Phonological representations are composed of a small number of primitive elements, using a few simple rules of combination. In some theories, the primitive elements are "phonemes," units roughly analogous to letters of the alphabet; in more modern theories, these units are further subdivided into "distinctive features" that specify things like place and manner of articulation; and according to some views, distinctive features are directly combined into structures such as the syllable. All theories of phonology supplement the set of primitive elements with a set of laws governing their combination, laws that express the redundancies of the description by predicting the distribution of some properties in terms of that of others. There is no general agreement whether there is one set of phonological primitives for all languages, but for any given language, an appropriate phonological description can be provided. Indeed, a number of competing descriptions can generally be provided, but luckily, divergences among various theories of phonology are quite irrelevant to the point I wish to make.

Why is such an exercise of any interest? After all, arbitrarily many descriptions of any set of facts are always possible, and the number of primitive symbols in which such descriptions are expressed can always be reduced in the direction of two. The short answer is that phonological descriptions are crucial to making sense of the facts of speech. It is worth devoting a few paragraphs to a brief account of why this is so.

If there were a meaningful level of description, intermediate between words and sounds, we would expect it to have certain properties. Call this level the P-level, and call descriptions proper to this level P-descriptions. We assume that every word can be given a P-description and that P-descriptions can be given an acoustic or articulatory interpretation, assuming appropriate settings for whatever additional non-P-level parameters are relevant. The sound of an individual utterance clearly depends on many things besides the P-descriptions of its constituent words (for example, the speaker's vocal tract characteristics, state of physiological arousal, degree of nasal congestion), but the contribution of a particular word to utterances that contain it is entirely defined by its P-description. This descriptive sufficiency should apply not only to all the existing words in the language but also to any new coinages, so that the notion "possible word of language X" is implicitly defined. We would expect that variations in the form of words, according to their circumstances of use, would be coherently expressed in terms of the categories implied by their P-descriptions. We would also expect that historical changes in the pronunciation of words would have a coherent P-level description.

Because phonological descriptions of spoken language seem to live up to such requirements, we can take them to be more than notational exercises. Humans seem disposed to learn, remember, and use words in terms of a phonological code; there is room for substantial disagreement as to how much of this code's substance is universal, but the obvious phonetic diversity of human speech should not blind us to the many consistencies and recurrences among phonological systems. Some simple, non-technical consistencies include (1) evidence for a syllabic structure, with phonetically sonorous vowels or vowellike elements at the center, and increasingly nonsonorous elements toward the periphery; (2) within such structurally defined categories, evidence for the arrangement of phonological possibilities into natural classes defined by features such as high/low, front/back, and voiced/voiceless. Note that I am not referring to the phonetic substrate for these consistencies, such as a jaw that can only open so far before it must close again or a larynx that can be manipulated to produce a buzz intermittently. Far be it from me to denigrate the jaw or the larynx, but my present point is that human speech seems invariably to be based on a conceptual scheme, a phonological system, in which the manipulation of the vocal organs is represented abstractly, in terms of simple structural combinations of a few featural primitives.

Some simple examples are in order. For many speakers of American English, a /t/ in word-final position has two systematically different realizations. When a vowel follows, the closure of the /t/ becomes quite short, and voicing continues throughout, as in the pronunciation of the phrase "at evening." This pronunciation is commonly known as a "flap." On the other hand, if a consonant follows, the /t/ is normally produced with glottal stricture, producing interrupted or irregular voicing, as in the phrase "at year's end." Such variation in pronunciation is usually called "allophonic variation." I have chosen a pair of examples in which the variation occurs across word boundaries and in which the conditioning of the variation requires a phonological characterization of the environment. To describe the regularity just observed (which is embedded in a larger pattern of consonant variation) we must use abstract terms like "consonant" and "vowel." No simple substitution of talk about jaw angles or vocal cord tension will do—the pattern simply makes no sense except when described at a suitable, that is, phonological, level. Examples of this kind are ubiquitous in human speech.

For a second example of the organizing power of phonological descriptions, consider the tonal patterns of the American Indian language Creek, as described in Haas (1977). According to Haas, in each Creek word one syllable has high tone (that is, a relatively high fundamental frequency), while all other syllables have low tone. The high-toned syllable is always either the last or next-to-last syllable of the word; the choice can always be predicted from the phonological shape of the word. Syllables in Creek are either open (ending with a vowel) or closed (ending with a consonant). The high tone will fall on whichever of the last two syllables is an even number of syllables from the last preceding closed syllable or, in the absence of closed syllables, from the beginning of the word.

Principles governing the assignment of stress and accent very often seem to involve such counting of binary units, interrupted by "heavy" syllables, and various phonologists (at least since Voegelin, 1935) have used such patterns as the basis of arguments about the nature of phonological structures. It is, of course, possible by such means to express the facts of Creek more elegantly than I have just done. My point, however, is that any statement of such regularities requires access to phonological constructs like "syllable" and description of fairly complex predicates over such constructs. Such cases are just as likely to arise in preliterate cultures as in literate ones and cannot be explained except in terms of a human propensity to define words in terms of a coherent phonological system rather than as arbitrarily distinct vocal noises.

If you will grant me the reality of phonological descriptions, what follows about biological autonomy? It may be that the need to have effective learning, recall, production, and perception of a very large vocabulary (given the nature of human memory, motor control, and acoustic perception) creates substantial functional pressure in the direction of a phonologylike system, based on "spelling" of lexical items in terms of simple arrangements of a small number of primitive elements. If this is so, it is reasonable to imagine that this pressure has resulted in some specialization for phonological learning, memory, production, and perception. On the other hand, if we believe that humans might just as well learn meaning units as arbitrarily distinct noises, then the ubiquitously phonological character of human speech can only be explained in terms of a predisposition that had some origin other than the needs of word learning and word transmission. For instance, it is not inconceivable that some system for sexual and social differentiation of cries provided an evolutionary substrate for the phonological systematization of language. In any event, there seems to be a prima facie case for biological specialization for phonology, linked to the large, expandable word sets previously mentioned.

Humanity's disposition to indulge in syntax is by some accounts even more remarkable than its bent for phonology. After all, the point of putting words together (euphony aside) is to express "ideas" or "concepts"; we may be prepared to believe that words are used to express pieces of complex concepts and should therefore be combined in structures that mirror the structures implicit in what they are intended to mean. These structures might be arrangements of systematic logical categories such as "predicate" and "argument," or might deal with categories idiosyncratic to particular semantic domains, like "threat," "supporting surface," and "instrument."

Instead, people insist on adopting normative patterns of word arrangement that depend heavily on categories like "preposition," "auxiliary," and "nominative case," whose meaning is at best either very complex or very obscure. As a rule, we can do pretty well at making out the drift of passages in which these patterns are degraded, absent, or constructed on unfamiliar principles. This ability makes it all the more striking that every human language nevertheless has normative syntactic principles of substantial subtlety and complexity.

It is not difficult to devise functional "explanations" for the existence of syntactic structures. For instance, we might speculate that the generation and comprehension of complex messages is facilitated by the existence of some set of structural principles and that conceptual structures are inappropriate for this role, say, because they involve too many interconnections to be easily encoded as markings on a string of spoken words. At best, however, such arguments can motivate pressures for the evolution of syntactic systems. As in the case of phonology, there is substantial room for argument about exactly what is universal in syntax and about how universal syntactic properties should be expressed and explained. But again, the regularity with which regularities recur—and the subtlety of the syntactic principles that normal humans master—makes it plausible that there is some biological specialization for this function. If there is strong functional pressure toward syntactic structure, then it is reasonable to suppose that evolution has followed along; if, on the other hand, the syntax of human spoken language is a quirk without any substantial communicative value, then we must assume it to be something like the biological equivalent of plumage. In either event, there is again a prima facie case for development of special propensities.

All aspects of language are constantly in flux. A language is constantly being reinvented by its users, who thereby express their identities as well as their ideas. Group identity is traditionally well marked by this method; all of us, like Liza Doolittle, signal a class, district, and sex whenever we speak. The fact that languages retain phonological and syntactic coherence under this constant reinvention is strong evidence for the everyday reality of such descriptions.

Other aspects of human culture also change, and the result is also the projection of various group identities through characteristics ranging from hairstyles and facial expressions to decorations on pottery or automobiles. Still, it is worth considering whether language may be in some ways "designed," or at least adapted, to be differentiated for such purposes.

The characteristics that I have mentioned are by no means the only aspects of linguistic descriptions that could be taken to imply cognitive autonomy. I have tried to take the strongest points and to express them in terms consistent with the widest variety of theoretical orientations. This is not out of opposition to theories or unwillingness to choose but simply because the differences seem genuinely irrelevant to what I take to be the strongest arguments for autonomy of langauge.

Notes

1. There are apparently reasons to think that evolution has redesigned this apparatus to fit its new function; see Krantz (1980) for a review.

A Psychological Approach   Z. W. Pylyshyn

Is language autonomous or is it just one aspect of general cognitive activity? To answer this question, we may apply a principle that has proved useful in examining a similar question that arises in the study of mental imagery: How does one distinguish commonsense reasoning from a special sort of "analog" processing occurring in mental imagery (Pylyshyn, 1981a)?

In analyzing what goes on in various types of cognitive processing, we must distinguish between processes whose regularity needs to be accounted for by hypothesizing *representations*, such as beliefs and goals, and processes whose regularity can be explained in terms of the intrinsic functional properties of underlying mechanisms. Most cognitive processes require both types of explanation, inasmuch as representation-governed processes presuppose a mechanism as well as representations, although the regularities cannot be captured in the latter kind of process without mentioning what is being represented. Thus, for example, to explain why a subject *agrees* with some proposition (where we are interested in explaining the agreement per se and not the words used to express it or the button-pressing response by which it might be indicated), we need to refer to a decision that the subject makes and to the knowledge from which agreement rationally follows. On the other hand, to explain the processes by which people access their mental lexicon (for example, in deciding whether some string of characters is a word), it suffices to provide a model of how the lexicon is structured and the access operations that are used because the access function behaves as if it were "wired in," that is, knowledge independent and not amenable to manipulation by rational processes.

But how do we know which type of process is at work—and is there a real difference? The view that the difference between these two forms of explanation is fundamental is described in Pylyshyn (1981b) and defended at length in Pylyshyn (1980). All we can do here is sketch a methodological principle that has been found useful in distinguishing when each of the two types of explanation is needed. The principle is called "cognitive penetrability." A process is said to be cognitively penetrable if its behavior is freely and rationally influenced by changes in collateral information—by changes in the subject's goals, beliefs, and tacit knowledge. This is not a precise statement, but it will do for now.

If we apply this criterion to language, we find that some language processing is cognitively penetrable and some is not. For example, take these two sentences:

1. The doctor did not rush to help the nurse because *she* needed the experience.

2. The doctor did not rush to help the nurse because *he* needed the experience.

What we understand the italicized pronoun to refer to must be explained in terms of world knowledge. Indeed, the weird effect of sentence 2 is evidence that what we know about the gender of doctors and nurses affects the processes that interpret pronouns. More generally, there is a holism evident in inferential systems—what happens in much of cognition may in principle be influenced by what you know. This closure of cognitively penetrable functions defines a cognitive system; with respect to sentences 1 and 2, comprehension relies on commonsense reasoning, not on some closed system such as the rules of grammar. Moreover, these processes requiring beliefs and goals are *not wired in*—they are changeable almost instantly by an informing context, that is, by providing information.

Since so much of our cognitive processing turns out on examination to be a species of commonsense reasoning (see Pylyshyn, 1981a), one is entitled to wonder what would happen if such reasoning processes were subtracted from all that is involved in language understanding. Would anything interesting be left? Now this is clearly an empirical question—there is no logical reason why language understanding should turn out to be one way or the other. Some processes—such as solving crossword puzzles perhaps or conducting criminal investigations—appear to involve almost entirely the general capacity to reason from world knowledge. Consequently it is of some significance that research in linguistics and psycholinguistics over the past fifteen or so years has shown that language comprehension involves processes that access an elaborate system of rules and other stored information and yet function in a way that appears to be quite encapsulated and independent of general world knowledge and the operation of commonsense reasoning. The process involved in using such rules to identify the logical structure of sentences appears to be autonomous and cognitively impenetrable and to operate independently of semantics or what we believe the sentences are about.

For example, one stage in the analysis of sentence structure involves identifying the lexical items that occur in the sentence. This process of accessing the mental lexicon, alluded to earlier, seems to be autonomous and cognitively impenetrable (this example is raised again in part IV). Another example is grammatical parsing. If we construe syntax in the appropriate technical way, the evidence from psycholinguistics (Forster, 1979) suggests that our beliefs about the world play no role in a major part of the on-line syntactic analysis of sentences. Our knowledge of syntactic structure appears to be encapsulated and does not interact with other knowledge in the course of parsing. That is what people mean when they say that language is autonomous—not that understanding language in general is somehow independent of our knowledge of what is being discussed but that there is an important part of the process that is *specific to language*, inasmuch as it is not just an instance of general common-sense reasoning, and that this part is autonomous.

A Neuropsychological Approach   H. Goodglass

The theme as stated—"Can we clearly distinguish language from cognition?"—and the approach taken by previous speakers imply that the question is, "How do cognitive and linguistic mechanisms interact?" I find that I can respond more easily to this question by considering the relation between the cognitive *capacity* and the linguistic *capacity* of an individual rather than dealing with how cognitive processes determine linguistic ones. In fact, merely by looking at how the levels of capacity in these domains are related, we can see remarkable independence as well as certain areas of relatedness.

We can distinguish between linguistic and cognitive capacities, first of all, in language acquisition. A severely cognitively impaired individual can learn the basic rules of phonology and syntax and master a great deal of lexicon. Of particular interest in this regard is the phenomenon of hyperlexia, found in certain children who, in spite of severe retardation, have a remarkable capacity to acquire the graphophonemic rule system of English, so that their oral-reading skill is well beyond the expectation for normal children of their age. A similar situation holds for certain patients with acquired brain damage; some of them have severely disturbed ability to understand language and to produce meaningful language yet are still able to read aloud fluently, though without any comprehension of what they are reading.

The effects of brain injury on previously normal adults provide further evidence of dissociations between nonverbal and verbal cognitive capacities. Many patients with severe language impairment have well-preserved cognitive ability in the visuospatial domain. Others have intact language but devastated cognition. But there is a catch in the interpretation of such dissociations: Any particular cognitive deficit may be due to damage in areas of the brain far removed from the left perisylvian region and may therefore have no bearing on the issue at all.

On the other hand, there are striking associations between linguistic and cognitive deficits. For example, immediate verbal memory is sharply decreased in almost all aphasic patients, and some kinds of conceptualization are inaccessible without verbal mediation. Even in operations that do not obviously involve verbal mediation, it has been shown that the concepts of many aphasics are impoverished in ways that do not seem related to their language deficits. For example, De Renzi and Spinnler (1967) describe the inability of aphasic patients to choose the color that goes with outline drawings of various objects that have distinctive colors, suggesting that the coherence of the concept, at least with respect to its color component, may be weakened. The weakening of the color attributes is only one example, but is almost certainly paralleled by the dropping away of other features of the concept.

Here again, interpretation is not easy, since the association might be mere accident. Thus abstract reasoning and conceptualization may demand integrity of the same territory of the brain that language occupies, so that their associated neuronal nets are independent but occupy the same volume of brain tissue. This would make it almost impossible to tell whether language and nonlinguistic thought processes are separable modules.

Nevertheless, it appears that phonology is separable, at least in terms of its mechanism of acquisition. Thus it seems reasonable to say that we can separate language from cognition at the level of the elementary linguistic skills. By contrast, syntax is almost certainly interdependent with cognitive skill because complicated syntactic arrangements are at the service of the intellect in the design of involved sentences. Moreover, with respect to the lexicon, there is ample evidence from studies of vocabulary size that word-storage ability is a close correlate of intellectual ability.

To answer briefly the question whether language is a coherent biological system—in the affirmative—I would like to point out that oral language may be some millions of years old. The perception and production of oral language become very closely attuned to each other early in normal language acquisition, and the two processes go on in roughly the same brain area. Written language for most of us seems to be parasitical on spoken language. In aphasia, the patient's written language tends to show the same systematic defects as does oral language. There are important qualifications to be made, with respect both to the congruence of written and oral language in the case of nonalphabetical languages and to their parallel impairment in the event of brain damage in the case of individuals who have very disparate symptomatologies in their oral and written languages. (We shall have more to say about this.)

Now to deal in more specific detail with the question whether phonology, syntax, and semantics are separable modules, that is, linguistic systems governing input and output equally on the basis of a single central representation. We see that aphasics can have modality-specific losses; in phonology, for example, input and output disorders are clearly separable. However, these do not look like disorders of a phonological rule system in either modality. Production defects look clinically like articulatory disorders, that is, disorders of control of the motor apparatus. They vary with the patient's oral agility, the familiarity of the target words, and the automaticity of word sequences. Many seem to be a product of articulatory mistiming. The only aspect of phonological errors that seems rule governed is the preservation of correct voicing, which is usually found when stop consonants are articulated in the wrong position. Perceptual difficulties in aphasia do not look as though they are systematically governed by phonological rules. Vowels and continuants are discriminated best; voice discrimination is maintained for consonants even when discrimination of the place of articulation is in error.

Thus defective operation in both the input and output modes of a "phonological module" seems, in fact, explicable in terms of relatively low-level acoustic and motor processes, not in terms of phonological rules.

Now I would like to consider the question whether grammar, in the sense of syntax and morphology, is a function of a central, or supramodal, representation. One fact that must be dealt with is that agrammatism seems not to be a completely unitary phenomenon. It is usually found in the patient with Broca's aphasia and generally involves both morphological and syntactic abilities. However, deficits in one or the other of these two components may predominate. For example, a patient may be able to produce complex sentences that are nevertheless impoverished in morphology (Miceli et al., 1981). As noted, writing often appears to be parasitical on spoken language, yet there are cases in which written syntax is spared in patients with agrammatic speech. This might move one to explain agrammatism as a disorder specific to an output system. On the other hand, agrammatism is sometimes shared by several different modalities (reading, writing, understanding), as would be predicted if it were a central disorder. Perhaps processing of content words, as opposed to the processing of function words, is solved by each modality in its own characteristic way.

We ought to pause here to consider the agrammatism of deep dyslexia, that is, the inability of the patient with deep dyslexia to read aloud correctly grammatical morphemes, free or bound. This may, in fact, prove a pseudoagrammatism involving special problems in the oral production of non-visualizable words, as opposed to content words, which are more concrete and more readily imaged.

Does agrammatism extend to auditory language processing? Zurif has shown that the usual patient with Broca's aphasia does not have normal syntactic comprehension. As a matter of fact, what is really unusual is to find an aphasic not impaired in comprehension of certain seemingly "simple" syntactic operations. But this is not true of all Broca's aphasics; there are cases where agrammatism is restricted to spoken output. However, as Zurif has remarked, this does not preclude a single, central representation of syntax, since input and output features might implement central representation in different ways. Moreover, when you do find input and output asymmetry, you may reasonably hope to find special lesion sites for the disorder. Finally, the fact that impaired comprehension is common to most aphasics need not militate against a unitary syntactic deficit in Broca's aphasia, since disruptions of syntactic input may arise from different lesions in different ways.

For example, von Stockert and Bader (1976) tested two cases, a Broca's aphasic and a Wernicke's aphasic, on a task that called for arranging words on written cards into grammatical sentences. The Wernicke's aphasic apparently could understand nothing that he read, but could place words in their proper order in sentences. The Broca's aphasic could read, at least at the level of carrying out simple written commands, but had difficulty putting words in an appropriate order in a sentence. However, the problem with interpreting these results is that difficulty with word order in simple sentences is not usually characteristic of agrammatic aphasics' production. This makes it hard to say what the relation is in agrammatism between the failure to order the cards and the production difficulty.

Finally, let us consider the lexicon. Here it is hard to imagine impairment being noncentral. Is it possible for a word to be understood without reference to a central store in which it is represented? It seems so. Comprehension of certain semantic classes of words can be selectively impaired while the output of these classes is normal. It is possible that even in the case of the lexicon, input and output may be detached from the central representation of word knowledge. (This will be discussed at greater length in part III).

In general, neurological injury may produce isolated disorders of phonological production, syntactic production, and lexical production. Isolated disorders of syntactic and lexical comprehension also occur. Whether a purely phonologically based breakdown in comprehension can occur is still open to conjecture. The perceptual phonological deficit observed in many brain-injured patients is problematic, since it may be quite unrelated to either auditory capacity or general language comprehension (Blumstein, Cooper, Zurif, and Caramazza, 1977; Baker, Blumstein, and Goodglass, 1981; Riedel, 1982). An exception is pure word deafness—which, however, may perhaps be accounted for by a prelinguistic auditory breakdown and should therefore not even be considered an aphasia.

PART II

Perceptual Processing Links to the Motor System

M. Studdert-Kennedy

The notion of a biologically determined link between input and output of an animal's communication system is a commonplace of ethology. Seventy years ago Huxley (1914) remarked that the courtship rituals of the great-crested grebe must have evolved by selection of perceptually salient patterns from the bird's repertoire of motorically possible gestures. More recently, behavioral geneticists have sought evidence of perceptuomotor genetic coupling in breeding studies of crickets and grasshoppers. The conclusion from several such studies over the past ten years is that generating and perceiving mechanisms are polygenically determined and mutually adapted, but not genetically coupled (Barlow, 1981).

The perceptuomotor relation is even more complicated in those animals, such as certain species of songbird, that have to learn their species' song. In such cases, the bird often seems to be endowed with an auditory template that permits it to select its own species song from the many others that it may hear (Marler and Peters, 1977). The template may be no more than a skeletal structure that gets filled out by exposure to a particular dialect. The bird then has to discover—by gradual development from subsong muttering to full song—the motor patterns necessary to reproduce that dialect.

The analogy with the human infant learning to speak is obvious. The parallel may be fruitful because a capacity for vocal imitation is quite rare—peculiar, it seems, to songbirds, certain marine mammals, and humans. Thus, imitation is a species-specific behavior that calls for a specialized relation between the products of perceptual analysis and corresponding motor controls. Here we should note that a child's reproduction of speech, though extraordinarily precise (as the persistence of dialects attests), is not mimicry; it differs from mynah bird or parrot imitations on two counts. First is the fact that, although the acoustic resemblance between a mynah bird's utterances and its human models may be remarkably close (Klatt and Stefanski, 1974), the two are produced in quite different ways. Nottebohm (personal communication) has described an African Gray Parrot who learned phrases in German, American English, and an Irish brogue, but showed no tendency (as would a human) to produce, say, an English phrase with a German accent. One reason for the difference is presumably that while the bird imitates speech (as it would a fire siren or a lawnmower) in analog fashion, the human divides speech into segments (consonants and vowels) for purposes of articulation.

Moreover, a phonetically identical reproduction of one speaker's utterance by another is usually quite different in acoustic structure from its model. Thus a young child who might, by appropriately·adjusting its vocal tract length, imitate at least the formant pattern of adult vowels quite accurately, does not do so. Rather, it automatically normalizes the adult model and scales its reproduction to its own vocal tract size and shape (Lieberman, 1980). In other words, a phonological system, that is, a *pattern of relations* among segments, is implicit in the child's speech from the first. All this argues that the motor organization of speech may be mediated by distinctive perceptual processes—in fact, by phonetic rather than general auditory perception.

What evidence do we have for the operation of such a distinctively phonetic mode of perception? And what can we say about its nature? From a variety of possible lines of evidence (Liberman and Studdert-Kennedy, 1978), let us briefly consider studies of (1) audiovisual adaptation and (2) duplex perception. The studies combine to demonstrate "on-line" perceptual dissociation of speech and sound.

Roberts and Summerfield (1981) started from a standard speech adaptation paradigm. In this paradigm listeners are asked to identify members of a synthetic speech continuum before and after prolonged exposure to (that is, adaptation with) a syllable drawn from one or other end of the continuum. If the synthetic continuum runs from, say, /bɛ/ to /dɛ/, with the boundary between the two phonemes set roughly in the middle, the effect of hearing several dozen repetitions of a particular syllable, say, /bɛ/, is to reduce the number of /bɛ/ responses and so shift the boundary toward the /bɛ/ end of the continuum. Adaptation with /dɛ/ shifts the boundary in the opposite direction toward /dɛ/.

The novel twist introduced by Roberts and Summerfield (1981) was to exploit an audiovisual effect discovered by McGurk and MacDonald (1976). McGurk (see also MacDonald and McGurk, 1978; Summerfield, 1979) showed that if subjects viewed a videotape of a face uttering one syllable, say /gɛ/, while listening to a loudspeaker play in synchrony a different syllable, say, /bɛ/, they often reported a percept different from either of the syllables presented — in this example, /dɛ/. Roberts and Summerfield used precisely this pairing (visual /gɛ/, auditory /bɛ) as an adapting stimulus on a /b–d/ synthetic continuum. Of their twelve subjects, six reported hearing the audiovisual adaptor most of the time as either /dɛ/ or /ðɛ/, four as /klɛ/, one as /flɛ/, one as /ma/. Not one reported hearing the auditory signal that was actually presented, namely, /bɛ/. Yet, for every one of the twelve, the effect of adaptation was that of /bɛ/ — a significant reduction in the number of /bɛ/ responses, and so a shift of the boundary toward the /bɛ/ end of the continuum. Thus despite each subject's conscious phonetic percept of an intraoral stop, his auditory system was appropriately adapted by the labial stop to which it had been exposed. The procedure effectively dissociated the perception of sound from the perception of speech, demonstrating that the phonetic percept is neither auditory nor visual, but abstract.

A second effect, dubbed "duplex perception" has been elaborated by A. M. Liberman and his colleagues (see, for example, Liberman, Isenberg, and Rakerd, 1981) on the basis of an effect discovered by Rand (1974): Two different percepts, one auditory, the other phonetic, arise simultaneously when the acoustic constituents of a synthetic syllable are separated and presented dichotically. Figure 1 displays a nine-step continuum of patterns sufficient to induce the effect.If the base (bottom left) is presented alone, it is usually heard as [da]; if one of the isolated transitions (bottom right) is presented alone, it is heard as a nonspeech "chirp." If the two patterns are presented dichotically in appropriate temporal alignment, the listener hears a fused syllable (either [da] or [ga], depending on which transition is presented) and, at the same time, a nonspeech chirp perceptually identical to the chirp heard in isolation. If, now, the patterns are presented for discrimination in pairs of stimuli, separated by three steps along the continuum, with instructions to attend on one series of trials to the speech percepts and on the other series of trials to the nonspeech chirps, the results are those of figure 2: For the nonspeech a more or less continuous function; for the speech, a discrimination function peaked at the phoneme boundary in the fashion typical of categorical perception. Once again, we have a dissociation of auditory and phonetic perception. (For a fuller discussion, see Studdert-Kennedy, 1982.)

The distinction between auditory and phonetic (or phonological) processes is not new (see, for example, Liberman, 1970). In fact, Donald Shankweiler and I concluded from

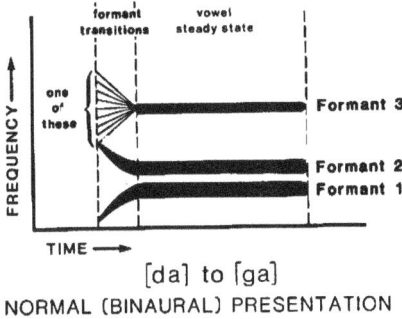

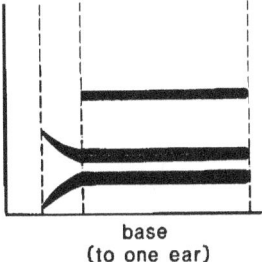

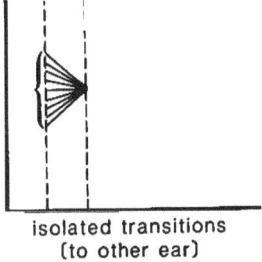

Figure 1.
Schematic representation of the stimulus patterns used to study the integration of formant transitions. (Liberman, Isenberg, and Rakerd, 1981)

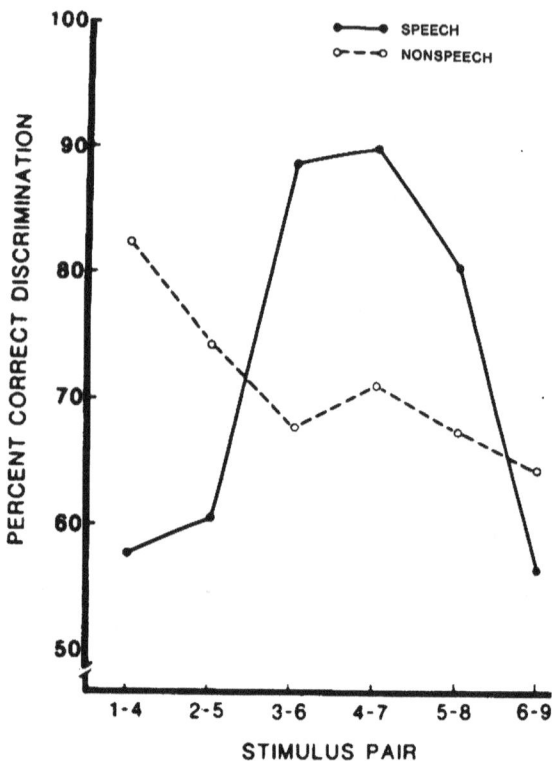

Figure 2.
Discriminability of formant transitions when on the speech side of the duplex percept, they supported perception of stop consonants, and on the nonspeech side, they were perceived as chirps. (Liberman, Isenberg, and Rakerd, 1981)

the results of a dichotic study over ten years ago that "while the general auditory system common to both hemispheres is equipped to extract the auditory parameters of a speech signal, the dominant hemisphere may be specialized for the extraction of linguistic features from those parameters" (Studdert-Kennedy and Shankweiler, 1970, p. 579). Subsequent work with normals and split-brain patients (some of it reviewed in the chapters by Moscovitch and by Zaidel) has tended to support this conclusion.

All that I want to do here is to raise the question of the function and possible origin of phonetic specialization. We do not know the form of a phonetic representation. Specifically we do not know how the representation is segmented — whether by syllables, phoneme-sized units, or features — but it presumably contains enough detailed information on temporal and structural relations among articulators to preserve properties of dialect. And this may provide a clue to phonetic function. For whatever the original function of dialect — whether to isolate breeding populations or to facilitate group cohesion within a territory — its biological depth is attested by the fact that every child does learn the dialect of its peers — and that this is the necessary route by which the child ultimately discovers the sound pattern, or phonology, of its language. We may surmise, then, that one function of the phonetic representation is to link the auditory structure of speech to its articulatory source. Thus the phonetic percept serves as the interface between sound and articulation.

This notion, in turn, offers a key to the origin and function of cerebral lateralization for language. The most striking property of the left hemisphere is, of course, that it alone can speak. If we add to this its dominance in manual praxis for some 90% of the population and the recent discovery of the linguistic status of American Sign Language, we may reasonably hypothesize that language was drawn to the left hemisphere because, first, that hemisphere already possessed the neural circuitry for coordination of fingers, wrists, and hands, adapted for tool use, and second, this was precisely the type of circuitry required for unilateral coordination of larynx, velum, tongue, jaw, and lips. The specialized perceptual processes, essential to imitation and acquisition (and, in due course, perhaps the neurological substrate of syntax) would then have emerged in close association with that fine motor capacity.

Comments

Geschwind took issue with the notion that the expressive aspects of language preceded the receptive aspects. He pointed out that if a mutation occurred making it possible for a human to speak, it would not be useful, since he would have no language to speak and no one to understand him if he spoke. The opposite side of the paradox is that if a mutation occurred so that a human could suddenly understand language, he would be confronted with a society in which no one was speaking. This form of paradox is common in the evolutionary study of any capacity that depends on linked activities between individuals. Darwin tended to approach such problems by looking for a series of evolutionary steps by which the linkage might have come about. The earlier steps in the evolutionary process may look quite different from the final product. It has been suggested that this paradox, although typically not faced by theorists of the evolution of language, can be resolved (Geschwind, 1964).

Consider as an example of one possible resolution of this paradox (of course, not necessarily the correct one) the following hypothetical series of evolutionary events. Let us assume that a distant ancestor of modern humans had some very limited capacity to associate the distinctive sounds made by a particular species of animal with its visual form: A mutation has occurred conferring this ability on some particular individual. This would be useful to him, since the characteristic sound of an animal would evoke its visual form, thus enabling him to avoid danger or to hunt more effectively. This would enhance his chances of survival and the chances of those to whom he transmitted the gene, and so this new trait would spread through the population. One could speculate that at some later date, one of the humans who had inherited this ability underwent a further mutation, enabling him to imitate the sounds of an animal. (This can be recognized as a refined form of the classical "bow-wow" theory of language evolution.) Since this new mutation would be useful, it too would spread through the population. From this point on, further specializations would take place, including, for example, those that would adapt auditory perceptual capacities in one hemisphere to the particular characteristics of sound produced by the human phonatory mechanism. The hypothesized hominid could now transmit information about an animal he had heard or seen to other members of the group carrying the mutated gene that made it possible for an auditory stimulus to evoke an associated visual form.

Although this particular hypothesis depicts only one of many possible scenarios, its assumptions are not unreasonable. In particular, it places emphasis on an ability underlying the capacity to learn names. It is often asserted that this type of associative capacity is widespread among infrahuman species, but this conclusion lacks experimental support. One perhaps unique study is that of Warden and Warner (1927), who found, on testing a dog who had been prominently featured in films, that he could carry out a long list of verbal commands (that is, *motor* responses to spoken words). His owner claimed that he understood many object names, but his performance in selecting the named objects from a group of objects was either at or only slightly above chance.

Geschwind pointed out that there can be forms of communication between animals that may seem to involve the comprehension of names, but do not, in fact, do so. Vervet monkeys, for example, communicate in the wild (Seyfarth,

Cheney, and Marler, 1980), but the hypothesis that the cries are *names* of specific predators, understood by other vervets, is probably incorrect. When one vervet emits the specific cry elicited by the sight of an eagle, the other vervets look up, but this need not represent comprehension of the name—it may simply be *a motor response of upward gaze* triggered by a specific stimulus. To use a simple analogy, the cry made on seeing an eagle may be "Look up!" rather than "Eagle!" It should be recalled that in the Warden and Warner experiments the dog showed evidence of comprehension of commands, but not of names.

Finally, the studies of sign-language acquisition by chimpanzees may not have represented the optimal strategy for research on precursors of language. It might have been better to study auditory language and to discover whether chimpanzees could learn the names of large numbers of classes of objects. This might have made better biological sense because of the known predominance of audition in language. Furthermore, Geschwind concluded, the stress on making the chimpanzee *produce* language may have been misplaced if the first evolutionary step was similar to that in the briefly conjectured scenario presented earlier.

Geschwind's general point concerning the problem posed for evolutionary theory by biologically determined behaviors linked across individuals is, of course, well taken: Human language is, in fact, simply one of a vast class of behaviors in which the activity of one organism is matched to that of another—from the food gathering of social insects to the hunting patterns of wolves and the mating of sexually dimorphic animals. Moreover, in communicative behaviors, it is perhaps futile to puzzle over whether sending or receiving came first, particularly since, as Geschwind implies, many small, interlocking mutations must underlie the behavioral complexes we now observe.

Nonetheless, the hypothesis that lateralized cerebral specialization for language was more strongly driven by cognitive

pressures for increased motor-phonetic range than for specialized processes of perception is attractive for several reasons. First, studies of aphasic and split-brain patients, as
well as a variety of experimental studies of normals (see the
chapters by Moscovitch and Zaidel), suggest that the right
hemisphere has at least some capacity for recognizing spoken
words, but is largely incapable of both speaking and the
perceptual phonetic segmentation apparently necessary (as
speech error data suggest) for speech motor control. Second,
the purely auditory perception of speech sounds seems to
be comfortably within the capacities of cats, dogs, and even
chinchillas (Kuhl and Miller, 1978), indicating that speech
is probably well matched to the general mammalian auditory
system. Third, on the assumption of some prior lateralization
for manual control, adapted to the use of tools, the hypothesis
goes some way toward rationalizing both the link between
handedness and speech and the similarities between spoken
and signed languages.

In any event, the issue, for whatever interest it may have,
is certainly not foreclosed. A telling question is perhaps
whether, in communicative behaviors, motor lateralization
does generally precede perceptual lateralization. Petersen et
al. (1978) have reported neural lateralization for the perception of species-specific vocalizations in Japanese macaques. But whether these animals also display motor
lateralization is not known.

Hierarchical Motor Control

J. C. Fentress

Two fundamental features of language that provide interesting points of comparison with animal movement patterns more generally are (a) sequential organization and (b) hierarchical organization. A third point of comparison is the genetic and developmental substrates of the sequential and hierarchical capacities.

As emphasized many years ago by Lashley (1951), the serial distribution of action—whether it be speaking, piano playing, or tying one's shoes—is a critical yet (still!) often neglected aspect of neural function. Stated briefly, the individual must be able both to articulate individual actions at particular times *and* to combine these actions into functionally coherent ensembles (complete phrases or sentences, a concert performance, or successful combination of shoe-tying movements). At a more subtle and sophisticated level is the organization of individual actions into variable combinations—such as using a given word in several different sentences. This is one definition of hierarchy in a descriptive sense (Fentress, 1976, 1982). It can also lead to the examination of neurobehavioral control (Fentress, 1980).

The idea of hierarchical control of sequences of animal behavior was popularized by Tinbergen (1951) at the same time as Lashley's influential writings. He did this within the basic framework according to which early phases of a behavior sequence, called "appetitive," provide rather broad rules of organization (for example, hunt for food), while later phases of the sequence are marked by the selection of specific acts tailored to the particular circumstances at hand (for example, large versus small prey). Tinbergen's model has been influential, though not without its critics. In particular, it is important to distinguish between the descriptive definitions of hierarchy (what is embedded within what) and implications about control (who is "boss of" whom) (Dawkins, 1976).

Early ethological models of behavior stressed the "innate" bases of many species-characteristic actions, though today it is recognized by most workers that genes and environment operate in necessary concert rather than independently (for example, Hebb, 1953; Bateson, 1976; Fentress, 1981a,b). In the long run this position may permit interesting comparisons between certain rules of development in animal behavior and the substrates of neural circuitry in human speech, since while studies of the former are giving more explicit acknowledgment to the various roles of experience, at least certain linguists have argued strongly for a species-specific foundation to human language (for example, Chomsky, 1980). (In a recent personal communication Chomsky was careful to emphasize his appreciation that environmental events—such as the availability of sufficient nutrients—are obviously critical to the development of the individual's linguistic and other capacities.) Nevertheless, at present most nature-nurture debates continue to generate more heat than light (Kent, 1981).

One needs to provide precise descriptions of ongoing and experimentally modified sequences of action before inferences about their control can be made. Further, it is important that these actions be described at several levels of organization, from the level of individual motor "acts" to the functional "contexts" within which these acts occur. At any one of these levels a basic decision of the investigator is where to draw the boundary between one event and another. In mammals this can be especially difficult, since several dimensions of action may be articulated concurrently, and with no obvious line of demarcation between them. (For example, how many notes are there in the howl of a wolf?)

Rodent grooming behavior has proved to be an excellent model system for studying these problems. The behavior occurs in predictable contexts (for example, in transitions between active and inactive states), is composed of a set of definable action components that are arranged at least descriptively in a hierarchical fashion (above definition), and can be examined from both genetic and developmental perspectives (see, for example, Fentress, 1972, 1980, 1981a,b, 1982).

The component structure of grooming in certain inbred mice is illustrated in figure 3. A key point is that while stochastic analyses, based on information theory, can give one an overall feel for the sequential organization of grooming, there are clearly places within this overall sequence at which the statistical rules of transition between individual elements change (that is, exhibit nonstationarity). It is thus possible to consider higher-order "units" of action that (a) are made up of different combinations of individual movement elements and (b) follow one another in predictable sequences. As illustration, in figure 3 individual "overhand" strokes (O) are found in units 1, 4, and 5, but only in unit 4 does a series of overhands follow one another in an uninterrupted sequence. Similarly, "Licking" (L) is seen in units 1, 2, and 5, but only in unit 2 do licking movements alternate more or less strictly with "circling" movements (C). While the mice do not always show all of the higher-order "units" in a grooming sequence (for example, they may start a sequence with unit 2 and/or terminate a sequence with units 3 or 4), the temporal ordering of these units is highly predictable (Fentress and Stilwell, 1973).

Interestingly, the "spelling" of these individual units (or "words") may vary from instance to instance while still being

GROOMING SERIES

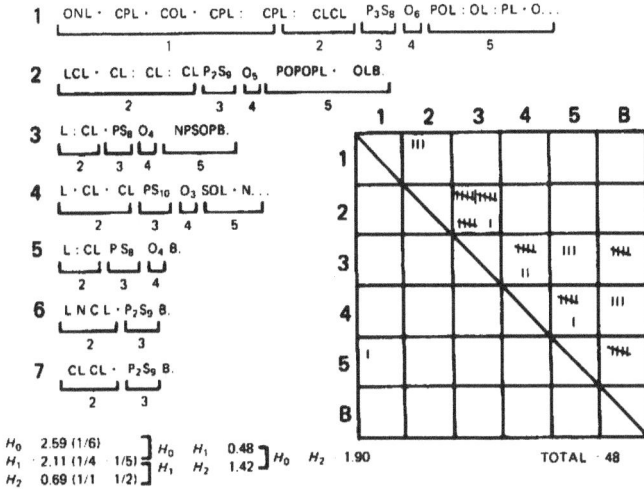

```
1   ONL ·  CPL ·  COL ·  CPL :    CPL :   CLCL    P₃S₈  O₆   POL : OL : PL · O . . .
    L_____J  L___J  L_J  L__J  L_____J
              1                    2     3   4          5

2   LCL ·  CL :  CL :  CL P₂S₉  O₅   POPOPL ·  OLB.
    L_____J  L____J  L_J  L_____J
           2            3    4      5

3   L :  CL · PS₈  O₄    NPSOPB.
    L__J L__J L_J  L_____J
     2    3   4       5

4   L · CL ·  CL  PS₁₀  O₃  SOL · N . . .
    L_____J  L____J  L_J  L_____J
        2         3     4        5

5   L :  CL  PS₈    O₄  B.
    L__J  L____J   L_J
     2      3       4

6   L N C L · P₂S₉  B.
    L_____J  L__J
         2        3

7   CL CL ·  P₂S₉  B.
    L_____J  L__J
        2        3
```

	1	2	3	4	5	B
1		III				
2			ʜʜ╫ʜ╫			
			ʜʜ I			
3					ʜʜ II	III	ʜʜ
4					ʜʜ I	III
5	I					ʜʜ
B						

H_0 2.59 (1/6)
H_1 2.11 (1/4 · 1/5) H_0 H_1 0.48 H_0 H_2 1.90
H_2 0.69 (1/1 · 1/2) H_1 H_2 1.42

TOTAL · 48

Figure 3.
Seven examples of grooming sequences in inbred mice (DBA/2J). Individual grooming movements are represented by letters, and their variable combination into higher-order units ("words") are represented by underlying numbers. While there is some variation in the "spelling of words," these higher units can be unambiguously recognized. They in turn follow one another in reasonably regular sequences ("phrases"), as shown in the transition matrix for 48 unit pairs. The numbers following H_0, H_1, and H_2 represent information-based statistics of the predictability of a given unit with (H_0) the assumptions of equal probability (therefore one could guess the next unit in a chain one out of six times), (H_1) knowledge of the probability distribution of units with no assumptions of sequential connection (one could now guess next unit one of four to five times), and (H_2) knowledge of the preceding unit (where probability of guessing the next unit is better than 50%). Differences between uncertainty estimates for H_0, H_1, and H_2 are expressed in log units ("bits") to the right. (Fentress and Stilwell, 1973)

easily recognized, and while the units themselves are strictly ordered in sequence. This implies several, partially independent, levels of control—some operating at the level of elements, some at the level of units, and so on. Preliminary experiments with neurologically mutant mice support this contention (see, for example, Fentress, 1972; Northup, 1977). At a still more refined level of description one can separate various measures within an element—such as velocity, area of face contacted, and so on (Woolridge, 1975). Here it is interesting that the data points are often more or less continuously distributed even though perceptually the observer has no difficulty distinguishing one element from another. This is rather analogous to the perception of phonetic segments in human speech, and it is important to decide how far mice actually do articulate discontinuous *combinations* of action even if the individual dimensions of which they are composed are relatively continuous.

In pursuing this problem it has been found that mice exhibit a phenomenon akin to coarticulation (assimilation) in human speech (Liberman and Studdert-Kennedy, 1978; Liberman, 1980; Studdert-Kennedy, 1976, 1981b). That is, the detailed form of a given action can be modified by its relation to other actions that precede and follow it in the overall sequence. This poses certain problems for thinking about elements of behavior as being discretely organized, as if by a series of neural "push buttons." Further comparisons to human speech may well reveal at least analogous problems of organization.

As a final note on the description of adult grooming patterns, invariances in performance may often be discerned at the level of *combinations* of movement rather than along individual dimensions. Thus a given (invariant) contact pathway between the forepaws and the face can be accomplished by variable combinations of head and arm movements, and a given trajectory of the forelimbs in space may be produced by variable combinations of movements defined for individual limb segments (Golani and Fentress, in progress). This implies that the constraints of nervous system operation may in a sense be "top-down," with individual features or dimensions being adjusted to provide a constancy of overall performance. In this sense, mice can also "say" the same thing in different ways. The proposition is akin to Lashley's "motor equivalence" and appears compatible with recent work on movement control where it is the *relations* between activity of muscle groups, for example, that often appear most basic to coordinated action (see, for example, Polit and Bizzi, 1979). The study of these *relational constancies* (Fentress, 1980, 1982) may well provide important keys to how the nervous system is able to generate flexible strategies such as are found at a more elaborate level in human language.

Here developmental studies have provided further insights. An initial question was whether mice master their performance of individual elements and/or units before they organize units into a broader sequence—rather like a child who speaks individual syllables or words before phrases or sentences. The data (figure 4) suggest a somewhat more subtle course of development. Individual grooming stroke types are often difficult to define unambiguously before the animals are about 10 days of age, but then emerge quite clearly with the help of supporting contextual cues (much as a parent may recognize the utterance /ba/ as referring to a "ball" rather than to the sound of a sheep, due to the context of the child's utterance). Once the individual units of action become adultlike in form, we begin to find evidence of their combination into higher-order units and of sequential ordering among these units as well. However, while the units may be recognizable, they still lack a fully adultlike form, and while they may be sequentially ordered, a wide variety of individual strokes is often interspersed. Occasionally one also gets the impression that as the young mouse is "attending to" the production of higher-order units and their sequential

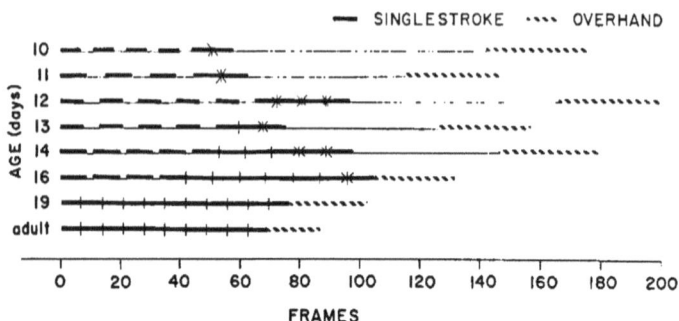

Figure 4.

Summary representation of single-stroke (unit 3) and overhand (unit 4) series in 10-day-old to adult mice filmed at 64 frames/ sec. In adult mice individual single strokes have a mean duration of 1/10 second each, are connected together in an uninterrupted sequence of approximately 10 strokes in which major and minor paw movements alternate strictly between left and right forepaws, and are then connected without pause to a series of overhands. In young mice there tend to be fewer single strokes in a series, the individual strokes are often separated by brief pauses (thin lines), there are occasional failures in left-right paw alternations between major and minor movements (indicated by ×), and there are often several interspersed strokes before the overhand series (indicated by gap)—although the basic sequence of unit 3–unit 4 is still evident. Between postnatal days 16 and 19 the adult form of the behavior is crystalized. (Fentress, 1978)

ordering, the performance of individual stroke types dete-
riorates momentarily—as when a child misarticulates a previously perfected word while struggling to put that word into
a more complex sequence (Menn, personal communication).
Not until approximately day 16 do the various levels of
motor organization within a grooming sequence appear firmly
crystalized—more or less all at once.

When one looks more closely at the coordination of individual limb movements in grooming, then various other
developmental changes can be discerned. For example, as
shown in figure 4, the strict bilateral alternation between
major and minor paw excursions shown by adult mice during
"single-stroke" (S) series in unit 3 is often absent in young
mice (shown by × in the figure); also unlike in the adults,
in young mice there are often pauses between individual
single strokes (marked by spaces between the heavy bars),
which can give the observer the mistaken impression that
the movements of young animals are themselves slower.

The latter observation emphasizes the importance of seek-
ing descriptions of the organization of movement from a
variety of perspectives and in an objective manner. Golani
and Fentress are completing a detailed analysis of the ontogeny of movement form and function through the use of
high-speed films and the Eshkol-Wachmann movement notation system (see, for example, Golani, 1976, 1981). To
initiate groominglike movements in mice from postnatal day
1, it proved useful to place them in an adultlike sitting posture
(figure 5A), a point to which we shall return. When this is
done, newborn mice (up until about 3 or 4 days) show many
elaborate groominglike sequences although contact between
the forepaws and face is largely fortuitous. These sequences
are then greatly simplified between postnatal days 4 and 7,
with stereotyped short contacts between the forepaws and
face. Subsequently (day 8 and beyond) the sequences are
reelaborated, recapturing much of the richness of phase I
while maintaining the precision of phase II. Again analogies

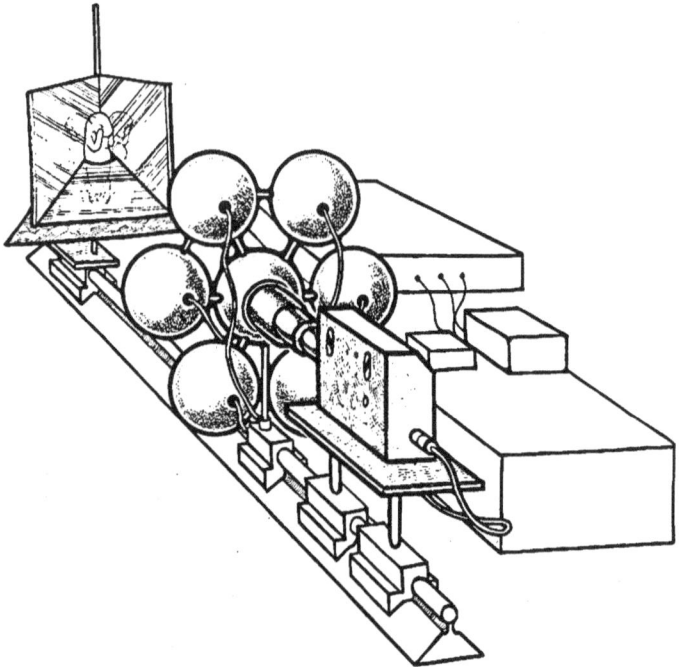

5A

Figure 5.
(*A*) Apparatus for filming infant mice at 100 frames/sec. using
stroboscopic illumination and mirrors that allow description of
grooming movements in orthogonal perspective. The lower mirror has a hole in it that permits support of the mice in a sitting
posture. Once in this posture infant mice can be made to groom
more or less at will (for example, by lightly pinching the tail).
(*B*) A globographic representation of grooming movements in a
3-day-old mouse in which asymmetries between right and left
forepaws and imperfect coordination of individual kinematics
within a forepaw can be seen. (Golani and Fentress)

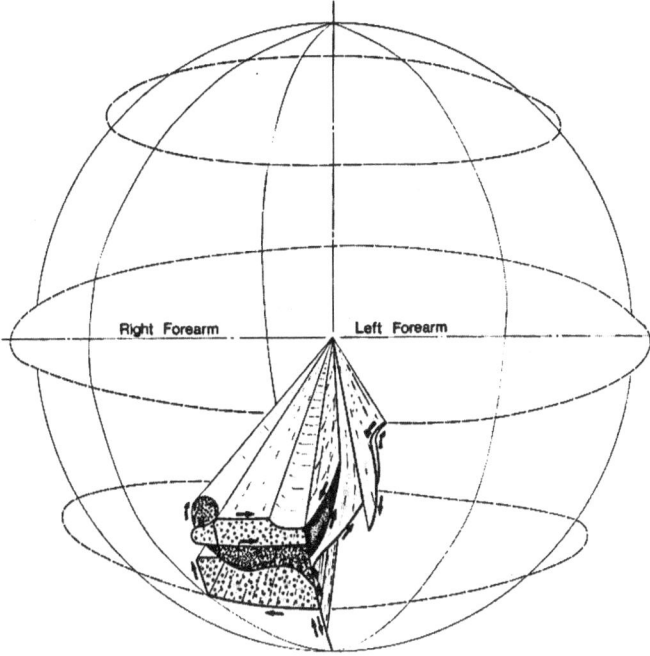

Right Forearm   Left Forearm

5B

are suggested to the sequence of language acquisition in children who often simplify their initial "babblings" and then reelaborate them—though, as always with such analogies, we should not infer common mechanisms (Fentress, 1981a,b).

An additional point of interest in the developmental elaboration of grooming sequences is the progressive improvement of coordination among limb segments. Two aspects of immature grooming relevant to the point are represented in figure 5B (Golani and Fentress, in preparation). This figure depicts in simplified form an actual grooming sequence in a three-day-old mouse. The two forelimbs are viewed as originating from a common point in the center of a sphere and from there tracing various trajectories along the inside surface of this sphere. The first feature to note is the marked asymmetry between the pathways traced by the right and left forelimbs; that is, observation of one limb trajectory is not a good predictor of the trajectory of the other limb. In adult mice the two limbs are usually coupled by easily specified rules. The second feature represented here in schematic form is that the coordination of kinematic details *within* a single limb is also imperfect in young mice. This can be seen in the pointed and "staircase" tracings, quite unlike those of adult mice, for whom smooth curves across the sphere's surface are characteristic. The importance of this for models of the development of movement is that one must deal with not only the progressive differentiation of movement components but also their progressive integration. A review of these problems in neurobehavioral development has recently been provided by Oppenheim (1981). Similar considerations clearly apply to language development as well (for example, differentiation of clearly articulated syllables or phonemes and their combination into words and so on), but the balance between differentiation and integrative processes in language needs further systematic study. Here animal models that focus upon the progressive coupling of intralimb and interlimb kinematics may offer interesting insights (see Bekoff, 1981; Fentress, 1981a,b, 1982).

In a review Kent (1981) notes that early speech production in children is marked by longer utterance durations, greater variability in form, and a more pronounced segmental structure (that is, lack of coarticulation) than that found in adults. Each of these facts parallels the observations made on grooming development in rodents. Further, Kent cites evidence that higher-order units (words) may be primary in the speech of children before phonemic elements are fully differentiated and that *both* growth and decay in phonetic articulation can be observed over time. Finally, as in the motor patterns of mice, the overall sequencing of speech elements develops before the precise timing of these elements as evaluated by adult criteria. Clearly, then, in both speech and nonspeech movements both differentiation and integration can be traced along multiple dimensions and at several levels of organization.

The reliable elicitation of groominglike movements from infant mice that have been placed in a sitting posture suggests that these immature animals may be organizing their behavior to a marked degree on the basis of "lower-order" sensorimotor cues of the moment rather than the more abstract "rules" that determine the behavior of adult animals (as when grooming is initiated during transitions between protracted bouts of locomotion and immobility). This hypothesis is supported by numerous related observations on unrestricted young animals; for example, they may suddenly break into a bout of grooming when the forepaws fortuitously pass near the face during imperfectly coordinated locomotor activity, or even while swimming! Similar phenomena can be seen in children (Fentress, unpublished); thus a child may suddenly leave its mother to play with a push-button toy, when the previous game of pointing to the mother's nose has led to a sudden loss of balance—and to an arm movement very much like that previously used to push the button on

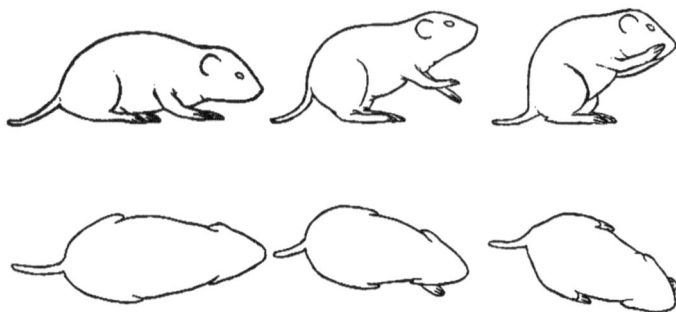

6A

Figure 6.
Two examples of "motor traps" in young mammals. (*A*) An infant rodent abruptly begins to groom when imperfectly coordinated locomotion brings a forepaw into fortuitous contact with the face. (*B*) A human infant suddenly switches to playing with a push-button toy when the movements used with this toy happen to be duplicated in a game with her mother. In each of these cases transitions between functionally distinct classes of action appear to be made more on the basis of movement "form" than through more abstract functionally coherent "meaning." (Fentress)

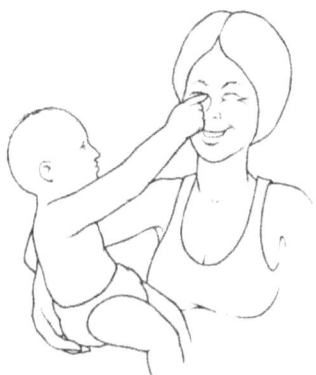

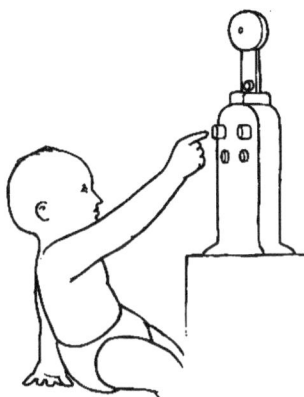

6B

the toy (figures 6A and 6B). Notebook records suggest that similar phenomena may underlie unexpected, and apparently arbitrary, transitions in the speech of young children. Words relevant to one context that are mispronounced to sound like words in another context (for example, /ba/ for "ball") may lead the child suddenly to leave a conversation about toys and go to a conversation about farm animals (sheep included) (personal observation).

While these data are preliminary, they do suggest a hierarchical maturation of movement organization, including speech. They find further support in behavioral profiles that accompany the disruption of higher cortical functions due to topical application of KCl on the cortices of adult mice; these applications are often followed by transitions between functional classes of behavior based on similarities of motor form (Fentress, 1977, 1981b, 1982). There are, moreover, suggestive clinical parallels with the speech of patients having various types of cortical damage. For example, Luria (1976) describes patients who generalize on the basis of phonemic similarities rather than semantic similarities (as most normal adults do). Thus if a normal adult is given a mild shock after the word "cat," subsequent galvanic skin responses in anticipation of shock can be elicited not only to repetitions of "cat" but also to semantically related terms, such as "dog" (that is, furry pets). Generalization to words that sound alike but are semantically disconnected (for example, "hat," "bat") is less pronounced. Patients with higher CNS damage, and also children, are more likely to generalize responses on the basis of sound rather than meaning. Sound represents form of movement as meaning represents functional class; if functional coherence in behavior is taken to reflect higher-order linkages of "meaning", then one can in principle devise methods to examine principles of hierarchical maturation, control, and the like. Thus careful analyses of hierarchically ordered movement patterns in animals may indeed reveal

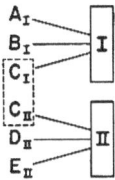

Figure 7.
A schematic summary of proposed hierarchical control processes hypothesized to account for the phenomenon of "motor traps" in young mammals (see figures 6A and 6B). Two functional units of behavior (I and II) are each visualized as containing several physically distinct actions (A_I, B_I, C_I and C_{II}, D_{II}, E_{II}). Further, certain actions may be similar for different functional classes (C_I and C_{II} in classes I and II, respectively). When a young mammal happens to articulate C_I in a form very similar to C_{II}, it may suddenly switch from class I to class II, including the subsequent articulation of D_{II}, E_{II}, and so on. This suggests that transitions in movement may occur on the basis of hierarchically lower-order connections in young mammals rather than higher-order functional packaging normally seen in adults. (Fentress)

rules of organization that are also applicable to properties of human speech, as summarized in figure 7.

The final issues to be raised are those of movement control and its development. For example, when adult mice are partially restricted in their movements (as by one limb joint being partially immobilized), they succeed in adjusting other components of movement so that functionally integrated grooming actions are maintained. This "conversation" among limb segments (and movement components in general) is often less perfect in young or CNS-damaged animals, again implying differences in levels of control. Progressive flexibility in behavioral strategies can be traced in this way (and obviously such flexibility is a necessary prerequisite to effect language use in man; see Kent, 1981).

An important potential limitation of comparisons between rodent grooming and analogous movement patterns in human language is that strategies in the former often develop remarkably normally in spite of severely restricted experience (see, for example, Fentress, 1973). However, it is worth emphasizing that, *in no case*, including the ontogeny of language, do we yet have a satisfactory account of the necessary interplay between genetic substrates and particular routes of experience—a point recently reemphasized, for example, by Chomsky (1980) in his attempt to account for apparent universals in the (grammatical) organization of language and by Kent (1981) in his examination of sensorimotor processes in the development of speech. Further explicit attention to these nature-nurture issues in a variety of forms of movement and at different levels of organization clearly represents an important avenue for future research.

Even the balance between central and peripheral mechanisms in movement control deserves much further analysis if previous static dichotomies are to be avoided. Thus in experiments with M. Woolridge (in preparation) it has been found that the extent to which ongoing grooming sequences are sensitive to modulation or disruption by changes in sensory (proprioceptive) cues depends in part upon the speed and stereotypy of grooming expression at any given moment. To complete the analogy, one may say that mice that talk very fast fail to listen (figure 8)!

To summarize, rodent grooming exhibits clear principles of sequential and hierarchical organization that are also hallmarks of human language production. The degree of flexibility in these nonlinguistic sequences is clearly much more limited than in language (mice do not appear able to articulate an infinite number of sequences with their forelimbs), but the very fact that nonlinguistic movement patterns provide simplified representations of rules that also appear to apply to language is an argument for future collaborative efforts among ethologists, psychologists, neurobiologists, and linguists.

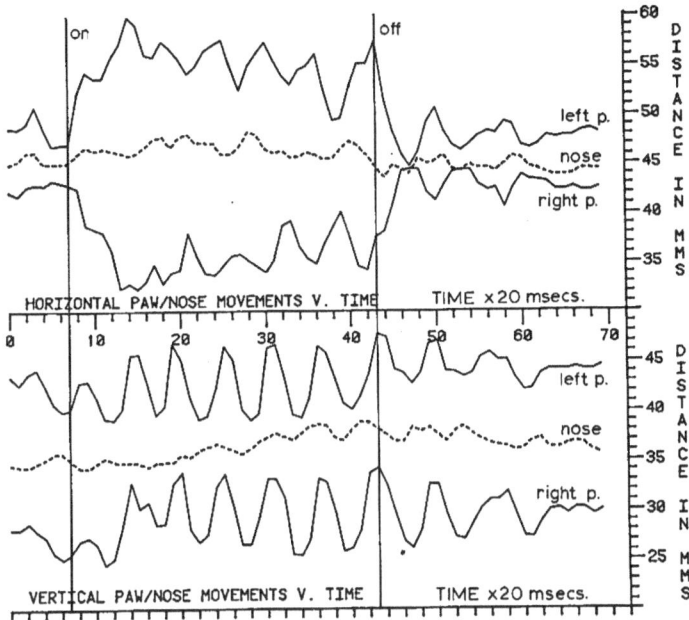

Figure 8.
Movements of each forepaw and nose of a mouse during a rapid ("single-stroke") grooming sequence viewed from above and the side. At the vertical line "on," the forepaws are suddenly pulled from the sides of the face via elastic threads connected to solenoids. At "off," the threads are relaxed. During rapid and stereotyped movement sequences, but not during slow and variable sequences, the animal continues to perform a full uninterrupted pattern of characteristic forepaw oscillations (but without contacting the face). Such data indicate that the relative importance of central and peripheral control mechanisms in integrated movement patterns can change in favor of central mechanisms during rapid action. (Woolridge and Fentress)

The problems of language—indeed the problems of movement control and neural action more generally—are fundamentally problems of "pieces and relations" in organized systems—in space, in time, and across varied levels of order. In language, in motor control, and in neuroscience we may have to move toward a more sophisticated bidirectionality in our thinking. For example, invariances at one level may result from combinatorial rules of variation at other levels, and while each level may be in some ways independent of the levels above and below, it may also in some ways act upon (constrain) those other levels of organization. Language—where what we say is partially constrained by our vocabulary and what we wish to say constrains in part the vocabulary we use at any given instance—reflects a bidirectionality that, one might suspect, is mirrored in many other forms of movement organization. It may be that our present inabilities to grapple with the full implications of the pieces-relations problem in neuroscience is, as much as any other single factor, restricting our conceptual progress. In this respect the detailed study of hierarchical organization in movement patterns less complex than language may provide insights that will be applicable to language as well—and to even broader ideas about brain-behavior relations (see Sperry, 1981).

Comments

The idea that language may be organized according to principles governing the organization of behavior in general is attractive because it promises insight into the evolution of language. Facial grooming in rodents as an example of a nonlinguistic behavior perhaps analogous to language is apt for several reasons. First, rodent grooming is an autonomous system, in the sense that it is a coherent, stable, phylogenetically ancient and endogenously controlled pattern of behavior. The pattern has not yet been subjected to genetic analysis, although its componential structure would lend itself to such work (Barlow, 1981, p. 239). Thus if grooming were composed of a series of *fixed* or *modal action patterns* (MAPs) (Barlow, 1977), we might expect hybridization of appropriate mouse strains to fractionate the system into its components. Breeding studies of cricket calls, for example, have demonstrated that a single trill pulse, produced by a single action potential in a single neuron, can be brought under genetic control (Bentley, 1971).

We would not expect to find a comparable degree of genetic specification in human speech, even if the experiments were possible. But it is conceivable that MAPs play a role in the ontogeny of speaking. Unfortunately there has been a bottleneck in the study of phonetic ontogeny for many years because we have lacked a framework for describing infants' prespeech movements and sounds. Recently, however, several studies (see, for example, Trevarthen, 1979) have begun to explore the possible contribution of prespeech oral movements and mimicry to the development of speech, while Stark (1980) and Oller (1980) have begun to supply the descriptive frame. Stark, for example, describes two separate sound-making systems in the infant: a "consonantal" system of stops, clicks, friction noises and trills associated with mouth constriction during the "management of nutrients," and a "vocalic" system of cries varying in quality, pitch, stress and rhythm, associated with mouth opening during the expression of distress. The precisely timed opening and closing of the mouth to form the syllable develops from the gradual marshaling and coordination of these disparate vegetative and expressive elements. More detailed description may eventually isolate and provide a full taxonomy of putative MAPs, or "articulatory templates,"from which the infant learns to shape the sounds that it hears. Such a set of prespeech movements would presumably be larger than the set of phonetic gestures observed in any particular language and might render moot the interest or validity of any list of supposedly universal phonetic features (see Ladefoged, 1980).

A second aspect of rodent grooming worth emphasizing is what Fentress terms the "relational constancies"—for many years a source of interest and puzzlement to students of speech (see, for example, MacNeilage, 1970). Golani (1981, p. 379) describes how a 10-day-old mouse pup, unable to move its left forelimb because it was displaced by the body of a sibling, nonetheless achieved descending contact of the left paw with the face by moving its rear limbs and shoulders, while simultaneously executing the normal grooming pattern with its right limb. Thus the usually symmetrical forelimb movements were decoupled and the MAP was modified to achieve the usual target of paw-to-face contact. There is an obvious analogy to the behavior of speakers who compensate for a jaw, immobilized by a bite-block clenched between the teeth, with increased raising of the tongue to achieve the target vocal tract area function required for a particular vowel (Lindblom and Sundberg, 1971; Lindblom, Lubker, and Gay, 1979). What is remarkable is that even the simple action patterns of mouse grooming are evidently not produced by central motor programs tied to specific effectors.

The third attractive aspect of rodent grooming as an analog of language is, of course, its hierarchical structure. Fentress describes the combination of isolated strokes ("phonemes") into higher-order units ("words") and the ordering of these units into sequences ("phrases"). The apparent analogy with the dual structure of language is striking. But it is worth seeing where the analogy breaks down, since it is precisely there that we may discover a peculiarity of language. Most obvious perhaps is that the higher-order units have no identifiable structure or function analogous to the syllabic structure or meaning of a word. As Dawkins (1976) remarks in a discussion of his own work on blowfly grooming, this does not mean that structures or functions might not be found, but it does lead to the further difficulty that, unless or until they are, the sequencing of higher-order units also has no apparent structure by which to justify the analogy with phrases. In fact, as Fentress shows in figure 3, the sequence of units is highly predictable as a simple Markov chain. Again, this does not mean that we might not be able to find in motor behavior an analog of phrase structure grammar—only that we do not have a clearly established one at present.

Biological Foundations of Language and Hemispheric Dominance

N. Geschwind

The term "biological foundations" is used here as a shorthand to represent the anatomy, chemistry, pharmacology, and genetics of the neural systems involved in language in the adult animal, as well as the development of the system in fetal life and childhood. The purpose of this type of study is not only to deepen our knowledge of language itself and its alterations after brain damage, but also—surprising to many—to develop animal models that might accelerate research considerably.

The notion that we need to know what language is before we ask where it is has little to justify it. The history of science has shown repeatedly that similar assertions about the necessity of knowing the "essence" of life, of consciousness, or of color vision have not stood up. One of the main reasons is that useful definitions frequently do not precede fruitful study but develop out of the results of research in many areas. The same may well be true for language. Since many hidden mechanisms may produce the same external behavior, it is only by penetrating to the foundation that we shall be able to distinguish what underlies a particular behavior in some special circumstance.

Although the content, that is, the specific language learned, is completely determined by the environment, the capacity to acquire language is biologically determined. The brain systems involved in language are delimited. Indeed, one should not speak about a contrast between language and general cognitive ability. All the evidence shows that the brain seems to have special-purpose computers for limited functions, and there is at present no evidence of any all-purpose computer. The existence of any general cognitive capacity must therefore still be regarded as questionable.

The language system includes structures both in the cortex and in subcortical regions. During development in childhood the cortical areas involved in language develop at different times. The region of the temporo-parieto-occipital junction is one of the last to mature and is also far more developed in the human than in other species. Another property of the language system is that it manifests dominance: One side of the brain, usually the left, is much more important than the other. The location of the language areas themselves is revealing. Since for the great majority of humans who have ever lived, language has come in through the ear and gone out through the mouth, it is not surprising that one major language region, Wernicke's area, lies near the primary auditory cortex, and another, Broca's area, lies near the representation of the movements of the muscles of speech in the precentral motor cortex. An important clue to the function of the temporo-parieto-occipital junction region is that it lies adjacent to the higher-order cortices of the auditory, visual, and somesthetic systems and is very likely involved in linking them (Geschwind, 1965).

We cannot separate out the basic biological components of language by studying only the *behavioral* manifestations of aphasia. It is necessary also to understand the anatomy. Thus in the syndrome of pure alexia *without* agraphia (Benson and Geschwind, 1969), the patient's only language deficit is in the understanding of written language. The first, seemingly obvious conclusion is that there is some specific group of nerve cells concerned only with written language comprehension. Study of the anatomy of the lesion shows that this is not correct. In the usual case there are two lesions, one involving the left visual cortex and the other involving the nerve fibers passing through the splenium, that is, the posterior end of the corpus callosum. Thus one lesion is entirely in nerve fibers and the other lesion involves a cortical region dedicated to rather elementary aspects of vision. Furthermore, neither lesion alone will produce the syndrome. The explanation (which cannot be expanded on here) is that the patient can see only those words that are presented in the left field and are therefore transmitted to the right visual cortex. Since the right hemisphere has, in most cases, only limited comprehension of language, the message must be transmitted back to the left hemisphere via the posterior end of the corpus callosum. A lesion in the latter location prevents the left hemisphere from receiving the message. This analysis has further consequences. If there is a lesion confined to the splenium, the patient should be able to read in the right visual field, but not in the left, although elementary vision is intact. This has now been documented several times. Note that we do not have to postulate a specific region devoted to reading only in the right visual field.

The behavior of the patient with pure alexia without agraphia is in many ways like that of a blind person who could previously read. Thus although the patient cannot read aloud or comprehend written language, he understands words that are spelled aloud to him, can spell words that are said to him, and can also read block letters traced with the fingers. In contrast, the syndrome of pure alexia *with* agraphia, in which the patient can neither read nor write, is a more convincing example of a lesion in a visual language-processing area. In the first place, the lesion is completely different from that of alexia *without* agraphia since it is in the region of the angular gyrus, can be confined to the cortex alone, and does not necessarily produce a field defect. This patient is indeed returned essentially to the state of illiteracy. He cannot read aloud or comprehend written language, cannot write, cannot spell or comprehend spelled words, and cannot read words written on the hands—all properties shared by illiterates. The point of this discussion is that without a knowledge of the structure of the nervous system, one could readily come to incorrect conclusions as to how the language systems of the brain are organized.

The apraxias also illustrate the fact that a *complete* understanding of disordered language performance after brain lesions cannot be achieved without knowledge of the nervous system. Patients with certain lesions in the left hemisphere fail to carry out certain kinds of commands, but carry out other types correctly (Geschwind, 1975). The preserved commands do not differ from the lost commands in length, age of acquisition, complexity, or linguistic structure. What characterizes them is that they are commands for axial movements, that is, movements of the eyes and movements in which the trunk is involved. This dissociation can be understood only from a knowledge of how the motor systems are organized. In these cases the lesions cut off the language areas from access to those parts of the motor system that lead to movements of parts of individual limbs or the cranial musculature (excluding the eyes). The language areas continue, however, to have access to nonpyramidal motor systems; these systems are distributed bilaterally and control only eye movements and coordinated movements of the trunk and limbs.

This phenomenon is instructive in another way. Obviously, the examination of this special class of axial movements, revealing the ability of the right hemisphere to understand and respond to a special category of verbal commands not defined by linguistic categories, was most likely to be carried out by those familiar with the structure of the nervous system, just as other types of useful research studies are most likely to be introduced by those with linguistic or psychological sophistication. Not surprisingly, since all published studies of callosal patients have used purely linguistic categories to test right-hemisphere language functions, they have failed to deal with this right-hemisphere capacity. In short, however powerful a purely linguistic analysis may be, it cannot account for *all* aspects of language performance any more than one can predict linguistic performance without knowledge of linguistics.

Let me turn next to a discussion of *cerebral dominance*. Until 1968 it was generally believed that there is no anatomical correlate of language dominance. Geschwind and Levitsky (1968), however, demonstrated that the area behind Heschl's gyrus on the upper surface of the left temporal lobe is larger in most people than the corresponding area on the other side. Galaburda, Sanides, and Geschwind (1978) demonstrated that this gross anatomical enlargement corresponds to a dramatic increase in size of an area of cortex of specific microscopic structure. The enlarged area is a portion of the temporal speech area of Wernicke. These studies demonstrated that there was not a simple dichotomy in size, but rather a continuous, skewed distribution ranging from many brains in which this area was larger on the left and a certain number in which the two sides were nearly equal to a smaller number that were larger on the right. In other words, there is enormous individual variation in the organization of the speech areas, and we must therefore be wary of the assumption that all brains are organized identically for language. Obviously, when we can identify the sizes of these areas on the left and right, in the living individual, it may be possible to determine whether there is concomitant variation in specific areas of linguistic competence.

An outgrowth of this study was the discovery by Galaburda and Kemper (1979) that the region normally larger on the left was formed abnormally in the brain of a childhood dyslexic; recently they have found a second dyslexic whose brain contains similar anomalies (personal communication). These disorders of cortical architecture result from abnormalities in the migration of neurons to form the language cortex of the left side, while the right hemisphere is quite normal. We thus have a situation similar to that of the visual cortex of the Siamese cat, which is known to be wired incorrectly; the dyslexic has an incorrectly wired language cortex.

This raises yet another problem: Disturbances of language acquisition cannot necessarily be analyzed on the assumption that the organization of language in the brains of patients is similar to that of normals because their brains may, in fact, be miswired. When brain lesions occur *in utero*, dramatic rewiring of the pattern of connections may occur, so that the adult brain is quite different from that of other animals (Goldman and Galkin, 1978). Standard modes of analysis based on normals may thus fail to penetrate to the fundamental core of these disorders. These new discoveries concerning dyslexia were an unexpected result of the study of the anatomical basis of fundamental aspects of the language system; they thus illustrate again the potential of basic biological studies for illuminating classical, but previously unresolved, problems. Many of the arguments concerning psychological motivation or bad education as the fundamental cause of most cases of severe dyslexia can now be dismissed. Furthermore, these new discoveries should enhance the possibilities of prevention and reeducation.

The final point relates to the common assumption that a lesion may remove some aspects of the language system and leave others intact; it is often thought that it is these intact remnants that characterize the language of the patient. This interpretation is probably often incorrect, since it implies that a lesion simply excises some part of the normal function. We know, however, that the brain changes after a lesion. The variety of such alterations is extensive, ranging all the way from very local changes, such as increased sensitivity to certain neurotransmitters; to much more distant effects, such as degeneration of nerve cells to which the damaged area is connected; and finally to even more dramatic alterations, such as the use of alternative pathways quite different from those used in the normal (Geschwind, 1974). The new alternative routes have very different properties from the normal pathways, however, so that although some degree of function may be restored, the normal state is not recovered. The language of such a patient may not consist of residues of normal language, therefore, but may, rather, reflect the use of other types of systems in an unusual way. Some caution is thus required in drawing conclusions from lesioned patients as to normal language processes unless one understands the subsequent neurological alterations, which, in addition, may themselves change over time. In some instances, one may be deceived by apparent recoveries, since the substitute function may, at first glance, appear very similar to what is seen in the normal.

Localization of   G. A. Ojemann
Common Cortex for
Motor Sequencing and
Phoneme Identification

This chapter reviews findings on the brain organization of
language, in particular, the relation between language and
motor system derived by Ojemann and his colleagues from
stimulation mapping of cortical functions during neurosurgical operations under local anesthesia. Application of an
electric current to the cortical surface outside of motor and
sensory areas in these alert patients disrupts actions, perceptions, and memories. The electrical stimulation acts like
a temporary, reversible lesion localized in space and time.

These studies implicate perisylvian cortex of the dominant
hemisphere in mediation of both orofacial movements and
phoneme decoding. The most posterior premotor region acts
as a final common pathway, and the areas peripheral to this
are sites common to sequencing of facial movements and
phoneme identification. This core area of the dominant
hemisphere is surrounded frontally, parietally, and temporally by cortex devoted to functions of short-term verbal
memory. In the regions between this memory system and
the perisylvian core one finds zones for specific abilities like
naming and syntax. These might be the sites for autonomous
pieces of the brain devoted to language subdivisions; see
figure 9.

The basic methodology by which these conclusions were
reached includes delivering electrical stimuli to cortical sites
concurrent with presentation of pictorial, auditory, or visual

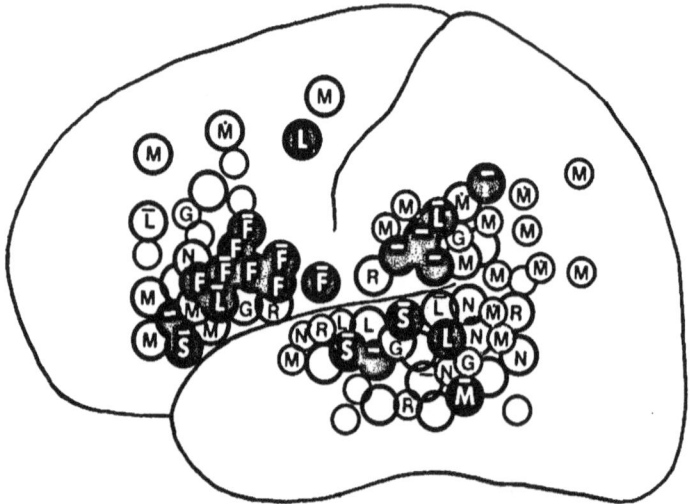

Figure 9.
Localization of changes evoked by stimulation mapping in a seven-patient series (Ojemann, 1980) during tests of the several language functions discussed in the text. Circles identify the sites where stimulation evoked statistically significant errors as follows: filled circles, errors in orofacial mimicry; F identifies final-output pathway sites with alterations in mimicry of even single movements; the remaining filled circles identify sites at which there were errors only in sequential orofacial mimicry; small horizontal bars, phoneme identification altered. Notice the congruence between the sites of these two alterations. N, only naming; black R and G, only reading; G, errors involve syntax (as defined in Ojemann and Mateer, 1979a); M, memory errors, the small dot identifying those sites with associated naming or reading errors; L, sites in which naming, reading, and short-term memory output were all altered, but not orofacial mimicry. The model of language organization derived from this mapping is discussed in the text. (Ojemann, 1981)

linguistic material. Test tasks include naming of an object, reading simple sentences, memory for the name of the object pictured, imitation of pictorially represented repeated facial movements, and series of movements and identification of a stop consonant embedded in a disyllable carrier /æCma/. In the last task, a list of alternatives is provided the subject, who then names the letter from the list of stop consonants.

A number of general conclusions can be drawn from these studies by correlating their results with those of more traditional studies of aphasic disturbance. (1) Some posterior inferior frontal lobe loci appear to be the final common path because transient stimulation there disrupts performance on every task, including all measures of language output and the ability to mimic even single movements. This is not face motor cortex, however, as no spontaneous face movements are evoked (Ojemann and Mateer, 1979a; Ojemann, 1981). (2) The ability to mimic sequential, but not repeated, single facial expressions is disrupted at more anterior sites within the frontal lobe and in more peripheral perisylvian cortex of superior temporal and parietal lobes. Phoneme decoding disruption is also found at these same sites. (3) Deficits in naming and/or reading are produced at nearly all these same perisylvian sites. These sites seem to correspond closely to the area that must be destroyed to produce a permanent motor aphasia (Mohr, 1976). And these sites are the likely anatomical substrate for the association of the inability to mimic facial movement and aphasic speech (Mateer and Kimura, 1977). (4) The sites where short-term memory is altered almost never overlap the motor-phoneme identification area, but rather surround it frontally, parietally, and temporally. Frontal sites related to short-term memory are particularly involved in memory retrieval, and temporal and parietal sites in memory storage (Ojemann, 1978; Ojemann and Mateer, 1979a; Ojemann, 1980). (5) Reading changes evoked at most loci involved nouns and verb stems. At a few sites only conjunctions, prepositions, and verb endings were altered during stimulation. These sites are interpreted as specific to syntax (Ojemann and Mateer, 1979a; Ojemann, 1980) and are located at the interface between the perisylvian motor-phoneme identification area and the area related to short-term verbal memory. (6) Clustered in the posterior temporal lobe are sites where evoked changes were confined to naming. (7) In all bilingual subjects tested to date, at least some dissociation has been found between the sites where naming of the same objects in each language is altered by stimulation. Two such cases are published in Ojemann and Whitaker (1978); a third case is reported by Ojemann (1981). (8) A semantic match test was also used, which requires, for example, that the subject choose the closest associate for *require* from *hope, necessity,* and *difference.* Subjects read the word to be matched correctly, but several sites have been identified in several patients where the only evoked change was that subjects missed the word to be chosen. These loci are also found in the area outside perisylvian core, frontally, posterior temporally, and parietally (Ojemann, unpublished data). (9) A hearing subject who knew how to finger spell had sites in the anterior temporal lobe in which only finger spelling was disrupted by stimulation. Resection of the area was required for clinical management of the patient's epileptic condition, and this resection produced a deficit, lasting more than four months, of finger-spelling production, even though other linguistic skills were intact (Mateer et al., 1982). (10) Stimulation of right-hemisphere areas have not disrupted these language functions when intracarotid sodium amytal testing revealed left-hemisphere dominance. (11) Ventrolateral left thalamus, a motor area, is implicated in anomia, a further example of common areas of the brain involved in motor and speech mechanisms (Ojemann, 1977, 1980).

Comments

Of the concerns Ojemann evokes, perhaps most important is the question of just how we are to interpret the evidence for any particular dissociation or lack of dissociation between functions observed under brain stimulation. For example, the lack of dissociation (that is, the correlation) between orofacial mimcry and phoneme identification certainly cannot be taken to imply a common mechanism for, or even a causal relation between, the two behaviors. For one thing, the stimulation technique may simply be too coarse to separate closely neighboring, yet independent, functions. But even if this were not so, we should be cautious in our interpretation of neurological findings in the absence of convergent support from other modes of analysis and experiment. As far as orofacial mimicry and phoneme perception are concerned, we have little convergent support beyond hints of possible developmental connections in studies of infant "prespeech" oral play (Trevarthen, 1979; compare Meltzoff and Moore, 1977; Field et al., 1982) and infant lipreading (Dodd, 1979; Kuhl and Meltzoff, 1982; MacKain et al., in press). These are not sufficiently well understood to provide a sound psychological basis for interpreting the stimulation data.

Similar caution is called for in our interpretation of dissociations of function observed under brain stimulation. For example, the dissociation between object naming and simple sentence reading has little meaning unless we have some hypothesis as to how the system is organized—neurologically, psychologically, and linguistically. Here we have an instance in which a sophisticated linguistic and psychological analysis of the behaviors involved might help to make sense of the localization data and to guide future stimulation studies.

Beyond these cautions, some skepticism was expressed concerning the whole notion of punctate cortical loci for punctate fragments of linguistic function. Are we witnessing the rise of "the new phrenology," from which we can expect to learn, shortly, the locus of, say, embedded relative clauses? The question is not merely rhetorical. For once we abandon holism and concede that isolated functions may be localized, we are committed to the question of where, if anywhere, we should expect the fragmentation to stop.

Finally, there is the puzzle of variability, both across individuals and across contexts. What can individual case studies tell us about the population as a whole? And what does the "on-line" performance of a patient under brain stimulation tell us about his "off-line" performance in a day-to-day situation?

All these issues are addressed by Ojemann in a later chapter on prospects for stimulation mapping during neurosurgical operations and in the following remarks.

Further Remarks on Stimulation Mapping:
G. A. Ojemann

Stimulation mapping is basically concerned with establishing relations between anatomy and function. The value of establishing such relations for the study of the neurobiology of language is twofold. First, they indicate at least some of the areas of brain that may be active during language. Presumably, since these sites are identified by errors in performance, these anatomical areas are crucial for the measured behavior. This technique would not identify areas acting during a behavior whose role is immediately subserved by other areas, for then no error occurs during stimulation and thus no relation is established. Once the crucial areas are identified, these become likely sites where physiological, anatomical, and chemical changes related to the behavior are to be found. One example of this use of stimulation mapping is the physiological changes related behaviorally and anatomically to silent naming reported by Fried, Ojemann, and Fetz (1981).

A second value of stimulation mapping is to suggest the role of a particular cortical site in a behavior by the pattern of changes (either dissociation or correlation) in various subdivisions of that behavior. Empirically, stimulation mapping often shows quite discrete changes in effects on different language-related behaviors, over distances as small as five millimeters (Ojemann, 1981). Of course, five millimeters, on the scale of neurons, are huge. Nontheless, this technique presently has a greater degree of resolution than any other for establishing anatomic correlates of human language. However much one would expect various language-related functions to be diffusely represented in cortex, these data indicate rather that they are discretely localized anatomically, at least so far as crucial ares are concerned. The identification of sites with changes in closed, but not open, class words that we have related to syntax (Ojemann and Mateer, 1979a) and of differential sites for naming in two languages (Ojemann and Whitaker, 1978) suggest that such localization may be surprisingly discrete not only anatomically but also behaviorally.

In the five different language-related behaviors we have examined, the general finding has been dissociation in sites of evoked changes (Ojemann and Mateer, 1979b; Ojemann, 1980). That is why the high degree of overlap between the sites where orofacial mimicry and phoneme identification are altered is unusual. Such sites are widely distributed frontally, parietally, and temporally. Thus if the stimulation mapping is too coarse to separate these functions, those separate sites must remain adjacent to each other in multiple brain areas, probably indicating a functional relation. There is nothing in the measures of these functions that would suggest that they should be related.

That these two seemingly unrelated functions, "nonverbal" motor mimicry and highly "verbal" phoneme identification, are altered from common cortex does not indicate why. Perhaps this reflects the anatomical site of mechanisms posited by motor theories of speech perception (see, for example, Liberman et al., 1967), but these changes could equally well reflect alterations in some mechanism common to both behaviors, such as temporal ordering of motor and sensory events (Efron, 1963) or fine timing mechanisms (Tallal and Newcombe, 1978). The concern is not whether there is an association, but that we do not infer a mechanism from the limited range of behaviors measured.

Subjects of these studies are undoubtedly an unusual population. There is substantial individual variability in the exact cortical sites with evoked changes in any one language function (Ojemann, 1979), but not particularly in the correlation or dissociation between different functions. Whether these are features of anatomical-functional relations in "normal" populations remains to be determined. The stimulation mapping studies suggest hypotheses to be tested in such populations, presumably by less invasive techniques, such as blood flow and metabolic measures.

PART III

The New Lexicon—A Summary of Some Arguments Pertaining to the Nature of Lexical Representations

D. Caplan

In these preliminary remarks I would like to illustrate some of the considerations that have led a number of linguists to the conclusion that lexical representations are more complex and detailed than was envisaged some ten or so years ago. There seem to be consequences of this complexity of lexical structures for both psycholinguistics and linguistic aphasiology that make it pertinent to consider here the nature of lexical representations.

In Chomsky (1965) the lexicon was a relatively simple component of a grammar, although its apparent simplicity no doubt hid an enormous complexity even within the terms of that theory. Roughly speaking, lexical representations were considered to be triplets of phonologocial, semantic, and syntactic information. Phonological information was, very roughly, considered to be the systematic phonemic representations of words along with phonological redundancy rules (Chomsky and Halle, 1968). Semantic representations have always been uncertain and controversial in linguistics, but at least some suggestions (Katz and Fodor, 1964) were available with respect to the nature of semantic representations in the lexicon. Syntactic information consisted of category information and subcategorization features, as well as a minimal number of lexical redundancy rules.

In Chomsky (1970) the role of the lexicon in word formation processes was greatly expanded. Chomsky argued that derived nominals such as *destruction*, were lexically related to, rather than transformationally derived from, their underlying verbs (*destroy*). The arguments are familiar, and I shall not go into them, but they have to do with the idiosyncratic nature of the semantic relation between derived nominals and their verbs, the lack of productivity of the process, and the natural way in which a new theory of categorization ($\bar{X}$ theory) would relate movement transformations, such as passive, around derived nominals and verbs in sentences. The theory of the lexicon was therefore greatly expanded because of the formal mechanism needed to express the syntactic relation between derived lexicals and their base verbs.

Since 1970, the theory of word formation has seen significant contributions from a number of authors, most notably Halle (1973), Jackendoff (1975), Aronoff (1976), Roeper and Siegel (1978), and Lieber (1980). In all these formulations, the formal structures associated with lexical representations and lexical processes have become richer. I shall not attempt to review the considerable contribution of such workers to the theory of word formation, but will concentrate rather on the nature of syntactic representations in the lexicon, an area which goes hand in hand with the enriched notion of word formation developed by these authors. In particular, I shall present a few positive arguments from Wasow (1977) and Bresnan (1980) arguing for an enriched syntactic aspect to lexical representations and processes.

Wasow (1977) sets out five criteria to distinguish lexical redundancy rules (called lexical transformations in subsequent work) from syntactic transformations. They are the following:

i. Transformations generate structures not in the base component of a grammar. Lexical redundancy rules can only move constituents into positions already defined for those constituents by the rules of the base syntax.

ii. Lexical redundancy rules can change category markings (for example, adjectives into nouns, and vice versa), as Chomsky (1970) suggested that syntactic transformations never do.

iii. Lexical rules are "local." For example, transformations can move constitutents over arbitrarily long distances, as in particle movement:

1. John called up his friend.
2. John called his friend up.
3. John called his friend of many years up.

There are, of course, performance limits on how far one is permitted to move a constituent, but within those limits, there is a "nonlocality" to transformations that is never found in lexical rules. Thus, Wasow considers that the elements that can be involved in a lexical rule have to be part of the thematic relations of a verb. In other authors, this local principle requires that no variables be stated in lexical redundancy rules (Roeper and Siegel, 1978), or that the items mentioned in a lexical redundancy rule refer to the strict subcategorization features of a lexical entry. Syntactic rules, by way of contrast, make use of variables.

iv. Transformations may be fed by other transformations, while lexical redundancy rules may not be fed by transformations.

v. Transformations arc more productive and express general regularities. Wasow maintains that within certain limits, transformations are exceptionless and that all idiosyncratic features of constituent movement are expressed by lexical redundancy rules. The idiosyncratic nature of lexical information is thus reflected in the nature of the syntactic operations associated with lexical entries.

vi. Roeper and Siegel (1978) add a sixth criterion. Transformations affect phrase structure nodes, while lexical rules affect lexical category nodes.

Considering these five criteria, Wasow gives several arguments that a variety of phenomena should be handled lexically rather than transformationally. I shall review very briefly his arguments for the existence of a lexical passive. This one example will then be taken up again with reference to Bresnan's (1980) treatment of the passive, which seeks to establish the existence of a sole passive that is lexical.

Wasow presents a number of arguments for the existence of a lexical passive, all of which establish that passive participles are adjectives, formed lexically rather than transformationally. I shall present two representative arguments. Further details can be found in Wasow's extensive paper.

Distributional facts indicate that passive participles occupy positions normally only occupied by adjectives. Thus, passive participles occur prenominally:

4. A broken jar sat on the table.

and in verbal complements of certain verbs, such as:

5. John seemed elated.

where no other verb form is permitted, but where an adjective is. This distribution is strong evidence that passive participles are marked as adjectives. By criterion (ii) that transformations do not change category, this marks the passive participle as lexically related to its underlying verb.

A second argument, both distributional *and* semantic, has to do with word formation from passive participles. The prefix *un* attaches to some verbs in both active and passive forms, such as

6. John unlocked the door.

7. The door was unlocked.

In general, *un* attaches to adjectives. It also attaches to certain passive participles, but not to the corresponding active form of the verbs. Thus there is no verb *unconcern*, but there is a passive participle *unconcerned*. The most economical way of capturing this distribution would be to consider certain verbs, such as *lock*, to be subject to affixation with a prefix, *un*, and to consider adjectives, including passive participles, also to be subject to affixation with a prefix, *un*. The idea that there are two prefixes, *un*, in English is strengthened by the subtle, but significant semantic difference between the verbal and adjectival forms. Thus in sentence (8)

8. The door was unlocked by the janitor.

the janitor actually reversed the state of affairs whereby the door was locked; that is, he actively undid a particular situation. However, in sentence (9),

9. The unlocked door was the third on the left.

there is no such implication of a reversal of action. This semantic difference suggests that there are two prefixes *un*, one of which attaches to adjectives, including passive participles, which therefore must be adjectives, and lexically formed, and a second, which attaches to passive verbs.

The conclusion is that there are two passives, one of which is lexically formed and one of which is transformationally formed. A wide variety of predictions regarding distributional and semantic features of these two forms supports Wasow's arguments.

Bresnan's paper takes the analysis of the lexically based passive transformation one step further, arguing that all passive forms are lexically produced. In her analysis, passive is an operation stated in terms of universal functional structure, according to which an item, marked as Subject, is deleted, and may reappear in an Oblique functional role, while a second item, marked as Object, is changed to a Subject functional role. This operation is accompanied by an effect on lexical form whereby the usual, language-specific, method of marking agents and themes is transferred from the original Subject to ultimate Oblique, and original Object to ultimate Subject noun phrases.

Bresnan argues that there are several advantages to this analysis. The first is that languages vary with respect to markers of agents and themes, and of oblique and subject cases. The passive always follows the markers established for these forms elsewhere in the language. There is an "illusion" of a movement in configurational languages, such as English, underlying the passive, but this apparent movement is simply the reflex of the fact that these case markings are marked by prepositional and word-order features of configurational languages like English.

The second advantage is that the passive form of the verb is lexically specified. In fact, the passive form of the verb is, in English, identical to the perfect participial form, and Bresnan's studies have not shown any languages in which the passive form of the verb is not lexically identified.

Furthermore, the passive participle undergoes rules of word formation. The arguments presented by Wasow indicate that the passive verbal form can become an adjective. Bresnan points out that it is not merely the form of the passive participle but also its passive meaning, which is incorporated into the adjectival form. Thus

10. The eaten dog

means the dog that was eaten, not the dog that has eaten. Since the perfect and passive participial forms are identical, the input to the word formation rule for the passive must be more than the morphological form and must include markings as to the passive semantic content of the participle.

This argument is strengthened by the requirement that the subject of passivized adjectives always be a theme. A very general statement can therefore be made: Any intransitive participle can be an adjective if its subject is a theme. This correctly predicts that there will be forms, such as *elapsed time* and *fallen leaves*, in which the subject is a theme and the passive participle is derived from an intransitive verb. This generalization falls out naturally within the lexical treatment of the passive by Bresnan.

This argument—that a simple statement of the generalization regarding the relation of themes to passive participles and that the word formation rules that generate passive participles must have as their input the semantic representations of the passive as well as their form—indicates that the rule for passive formation is lexical rather than transformational.

Bresnan presents a variety of other arguments in support of her position. She argues that verbal compounds (such as *dishwashing machine*) are also a source of evidence for the existence of lexical rules of word formation that take as input the passive forms. She deals with a number of problems in her analysis, in particular, the interaction of passive with movement transformations, such as raising to object position and equi-noun-phrase deletion. Details of the arguments can be found in her paper.

I have presented a few arguments to indicate that features of syntactic form previously thought to be associated with the transformational component of a grammar can be reconsidered as lexical processes. I have not presented counterarguments and have not attempted to go into the detail of the analyses or to present areas in which they are unsatisfactory. The main purpose of this sketchy presentation is to indicate that even in the realm of syntax, and certainly in the realm of word formation, phonology, and semantics, our notions of the lexicon are changing in a way that increases the complexity of lexical representations and the power of linguistic operations associated with lexical entries. I shall conclude by briefly mentioning some of the possible consequences of this view for psycholinguistic and neurolinguistic work.

In the area of psycholinguistics and language processing, it is clear that if this kind of information is arrayed against lexical items, then lexical access may reveal a great deal more about what we take to be the syntactic structure of an utterance than had previously been thought. This might be important in terms of production and perception routines. If, to take one example, lexical access from bottom-up information in sentence perception includes a great deal of syntactic information arrayed against lexical items, one might expect that parsing routines would look very different from those suggested by, for example, Thorne, Bradley, and Dewar (1968), which derive a great deal of syntactic information from analysis of the closed-class vocabulary. The same may be true for speech production and for the processes of language acquisition.

In the area of neurolinguistics, concerning the performance of patients who have breakdown of language due to cerebral lesions and other causes, a roughly comparable set of observations can be made. On the one hand, if loss of access to major lexical items entails loss of access to a rich set of linguistic representations, we might expect such loss of access to involve more consequences for what are superficially apparent as syntactic abilities than had been previously considered. On the other hand, if access to major lexical items is retained, as may be the case in agrammatism, many more syntactic structures may be available to patients than had previously been thought. This theme is treated in my later chapter on agrammatism.

Clearly, then, one important challenge for aphasiology and for the psychology of language is to consider the possibility of a rich lexicon and to develop a taxonomy of lexical structures and operations relevant to language use and breakdown.

Comments

Mark Liberman pointed out that the work just described may be seen as part of a broader movement that has been taking place in linguistic theory for several years. Many linguists are abandoning the assumption of early work in transformational grammar that surface-structure regularities are epiphenomenal, that is, the accidental products of deeper regularities. They are returning to the more commonsense view that the immediate constituent structure, evident in the sequence of words in a sentence, rather closely represents the important regularities of the system.

Nonetheless, this may not be easy. Even in a word-order language, such as English, one cannot always read off directly from the surface structure of the sentence who did what to whom. In fact, one of the important jobs for transformations used to be precisely to restore the predicate-argument structure to a form as clear as it would have in the predicate calculus.

Finally, we should remember that there are many equivalent ways of providing a formal description of a language. Therefore, when we come to apply such descriptions in other domains, we should not be constrained by the formalisms that happen to be available (because some one happens to have done the work in a particular area). Rather, we should see the whole gamut of descriptions (including the work just discussed) as simply enriching the alternatives that may, or may not, throw light when applied in other domains of study.

Stages of Processing and Hemispheric Differences in Language in the Normal Subject

M. Moscovitch

Does the right hemisphere contribute to language function in normal right-handed people? We know that aphasic patients with left-hemisphere lesion may sometimes retain certain functions, particularly semantic ones. Broca's aphasics may be relatively more impaired syntactically than semantically (Caramazza and Berndt, 1978; Goodglass, 1968; Schwartz, Saffran, and Marin, 1980; Zurif et al., 1974), and individuals with phonemic or deep dyslexia as a result of left-hemisphere lesions have difficulty reading phonetically, but are less impaired in extracting meaning via another route from script (Coltheart, 1980; Marshall and Newcombe, 1973). In both of these syndromes, investigators suspect that the right hemisphere may be performing the linguistic functions observed, although at the moment there is little evidence to back this up (Coltheart, 1980; Critchley, 1962; Czopf, 1972; Gowers, 1887; Kinsbourne, 1971; Moscovitch, 1976, 1982; Neilson, 1946; Russel and Espir, 1961; Saffran, Schwartz, and Marin, 1980; Searlman, 1978; Zangwill, 1960). The linguistic activities of the right hemisphere have also been investigated in patients who have undergone hemispherectomy and commissurotomy. As expected from the aphasia literature, simple syntactic functions are preserved in some, but by no means the majority of the patients (for summaries see Dennis, 1980; Gazzaniga, 1970; Gazzaniga and LeDoux, 1978; Moscovitch, 1981; Searlman, 1977; Zaidel, 1978a,b,c). Their semantic systems, as assessed by comprehension and production of single words and sentences, however, seem less impaired. If, as these studies suggest, the right hemisphere has a rich lexicon, does its organization mimic that of the normal left hemisphere, and does it make a contribution to normal linguistic performance that is commensurate with its semantic capacity? To answer these questions, we need to examine the linguistic performances of normal people and of people with right-hemisphere damage.

Despite severe limitations in the techniques available to study hemispheric differences in normal people, definite progress has been made. Research in both audition and vision has generally supported findings from the clinical literature that hemispheric asymmetries are found primarily at later, higher-order stages of information processing (for recent reviews see Berlin and McNeil, 1976; Moscovitch, 1979; Madden and Nebes, 1980; and Bradshaw and Nettleton, 1981; and for a dissenting view see Kimura and Durnford, 1974). Recent studies with visual masking techniques have further supported this position (Hellige and Cox, 1976; Moscovitch, Scullion, and Christie, 1976; Proudfoot, 1982; McKeeves and Suberi, 1974). In our laboratory, three-letter words arranged vertically were presented tachistoscopically for durations ranging from 2 to 16 milliseconds to either the right or left visual field, followed, after interstimulus intervals (ISI) of 2–24 milliseconds by either a flash or pattern mask. The subject's task was to identify the word. As the ISI between the target and mask was increased, identification improved until it reached a criterion of four consecutive correct responses. The ISI value at this level of performance was taken as the *critical ISI*. Because the flash mask is effective only when it is presented to the same eye as the target, it is considered to act peripherally (Turvey, 1973). The pattern mask is effective even when it is presented to the eye opposite the target and is consequently assumed to act centrally at, or beyond, the point at which input from the two eyes converge (Turvey, 1973). If hemispheric asymmetries arise at later processing stages but are absent at very early ones, we should find perceptual asymmetries only in the pattern-masking condition. As predicted, the critical ISI at which the target escaped the mask was shorter in the right field-left hemisphere only in the pattern mask condition. In the flash mask condition, no hemi-field differences were noted (see figure 10).

A subsequent study conducted in collaboration with Mark Byrd confirmed these results. Because critical ISI is a measure of performance at only one point in the identification function, we decided to look at accuracy of target identification at different stimulus onset asynchronies (SOA) between the target and the mask. It might have been the case, for example, that at low SOAs, identification, though poor, favored one visual field, whereas at higher SOAs, as identification improved, performance favored the opposite field. As before, subjects were presented with a vertical three-letter target followed by a flash (visual noise) or pattern mask at different SOAs. As figure 11 shows, a large and consistent advantage in favor of the right field-left hemisphere was evident only in the pattern-mask condition. Significantly, this advantage appeared as soon as any identification was possible and was maintained virtually unchanged at all subsequent SOAs.

A clue to the structural locus at which these asymmetries first appear comes from masking studies that Schlotterer, Crapper, and I conducted on patients suffering from senile dementia of the Alzheimer type (Schlotterer, 1977; Schlotterer, Moscovitch, and MacLachlan, submitted for publication). We found that compared to age-matched controls and young normal subjects, Alzheimer patients showed a marked decrement in identification of a foveally presented letter in the pattern-mask condition relative to that of the flash mask, where performance was indistinguishable from normal. The SOA at which identification was perfect in the pattern mask condition was over 75 milliseconds longer in

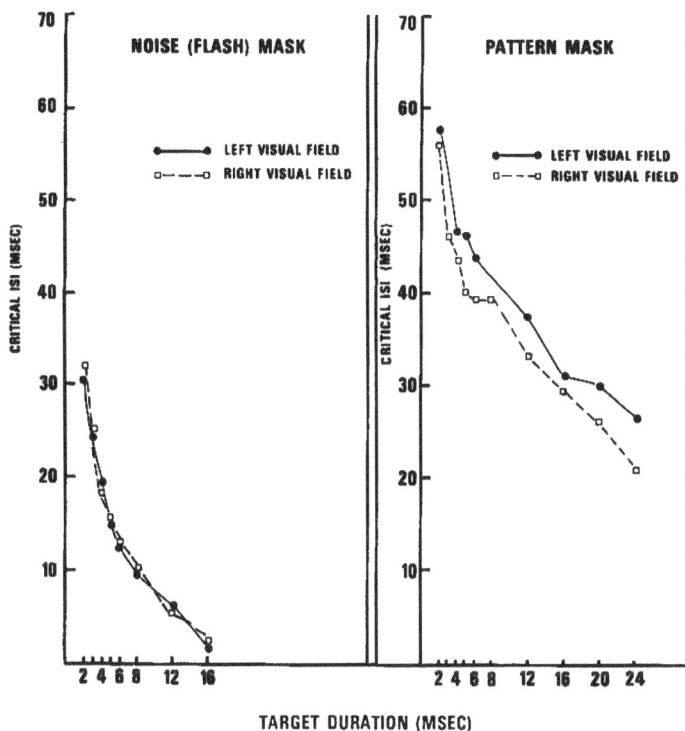

Figure 10.
Relation between target duration and mean critical interstimulus interval (ISI) for masking by noise and pattern (50-msec duration) when the target and mask appear in the same visual field. The target is a three-letter word presented vertically. (Moscovitch, 1979)

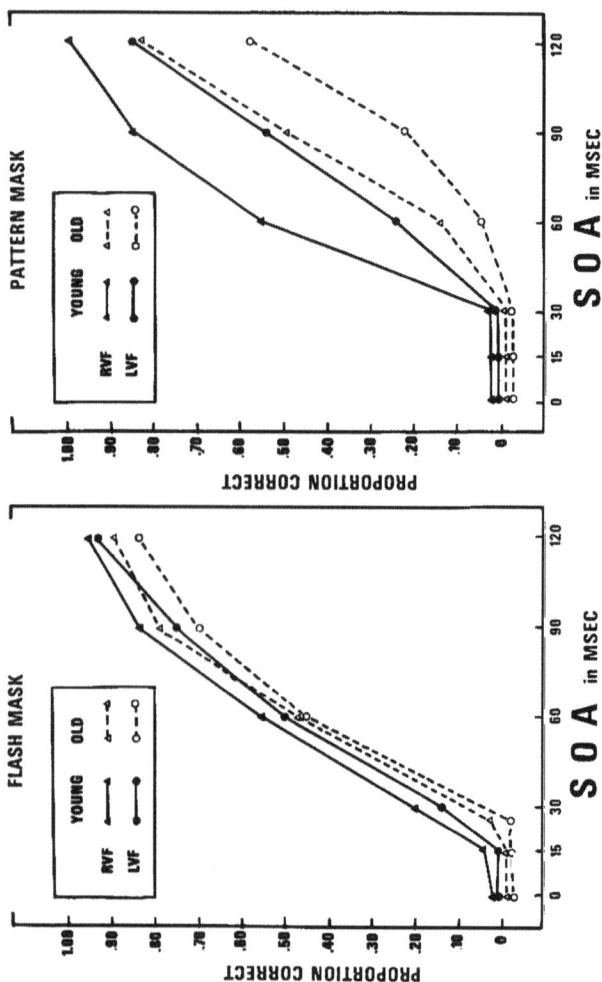

Figure 11.
Proportions of correct identifications by young (under 30) and old (over 65) people of a three-letter target presented in the right or left visual field for a duration of 2 msec. The mask was either a flash or a pattern that was presented for a duration of 50 msec in both fields at varying stimulus onset asynchronies (SOAs) from the target. (Moscovitch)

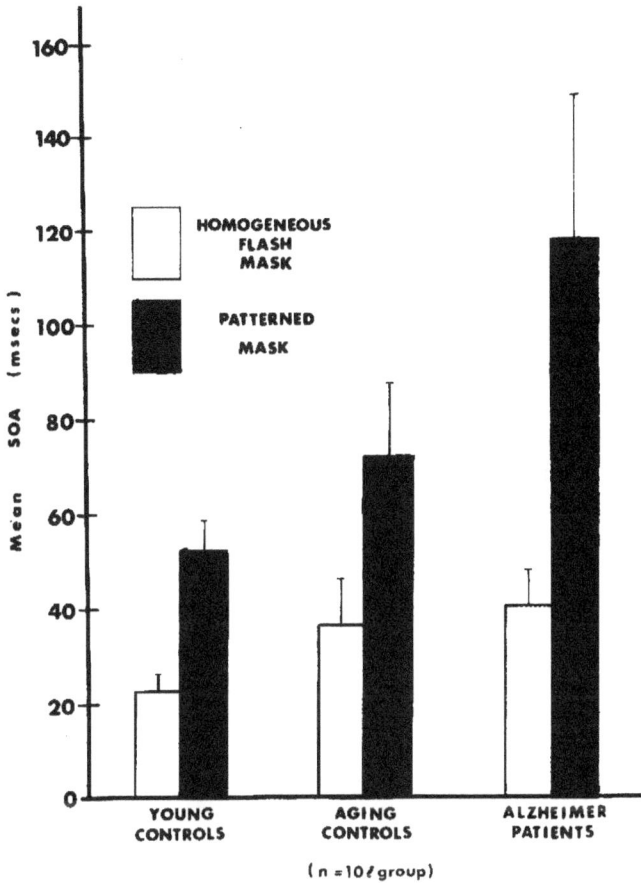

Figure 12.
Mean vertical stimulus onset asynchrony (SOA) between target and mask at which a foveally presented single-letter target is identified correctly on four successive trials. The mask was either a flash or a pattern of 50-msec duration that was superimposed on the target. (Moscovitch)

Alzheimer patients than in controls (figure 12). Because the degenerative changes characteristic of Alzheimer's disease, such as the presence of neurofibrillary tangles and senile placques, are relatively rare posterior to striate cortex, but proliferate in areas anterior to it, such as the prestriate and temporal lobes (Tomlinson, Blessed, and Roth, 1970), these results suggest that the pattern mask acts anterior to striate cortex. The Alzheimer's patients' normal performance on the flash-mask condition is consistent with the fact that it is a more peripheral process that may be handled by the relatively intact structures of their visual system.

Beyond the early stages, from both functional and structural points of view, information is processed differently by the two hemispheres (figure 13). This applies to all kinds of information or types of stimulus input. Where hemispheric differences are large, as in processing syntactic or phonological properties of language, one can assume that the inferior hemisphere's capacities are simply inadequate or inappropriate to the task. In many instances, however, as in processing semantic properties of language or in classifying objects and interpreting events, hemispheric differences, measured in absolute performance levels, are likely to be smaller because each hemisphere contributes in its own way to the task at hand.

These observations regarding large hemispheric differences in performance are derived primarily from clinical populations. In testing for hemispheric specialization in normal people, one is limited to studying perceptual or motor asymmetries that are small even when they are presumed to reflect large differences between the cerebral hemispheres. It could not be otherwise, given the interconnections of an intact brain and the speed of neural transmission. Thus it is assumed that a consistent advantage in stimulus recognition of 30 milliseconds in latency or 10 percent in accuracy for one visual field (or ear) over the other indicates that the hemisphere contralateral to the favored field (or ear) is the dom-

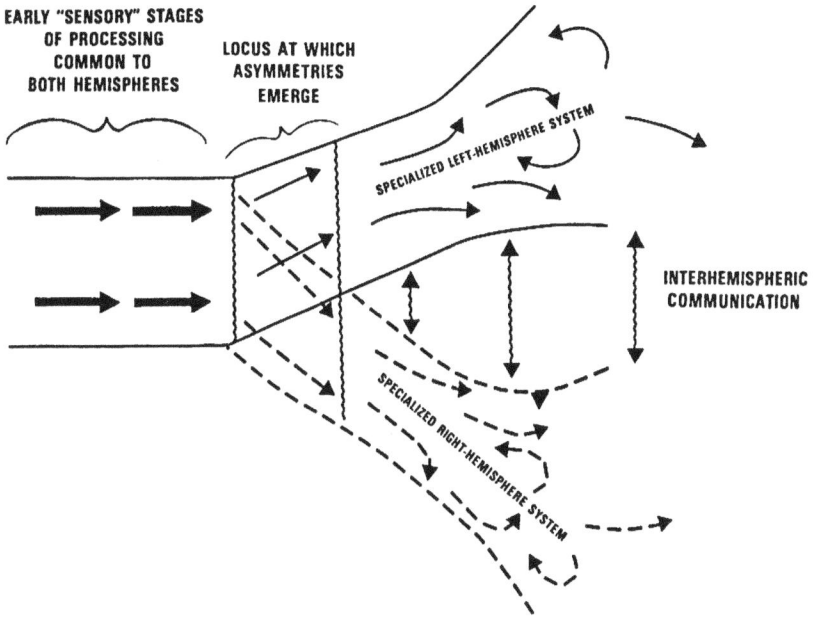

EARLY "SENSORY" STAGES
OF PROCESSING
COMMON TO
BOTH HEMISPHERES

LOCUS AT WHICH
ASYMMETRIES
EMERGE

SPECIALIZED LEFT-HEMISPHERE SYSTEM

SPECIALIZED RIGHT-HEMISPHERE SYSTEM

INTERHEMISPHERIC
COMMUNICATION

Figure 13.
Model of information flow according to the transmitted lateralization
hypothesis.

inant one performing the task. Unfortunately, even these differences are often fragile, in that a variety of attentional factors can bias performance toward or away from a given sensory field.

Despite these drawbacks, some reaction-time (RT) techniques have been devised that are relatively resistant to these performance variables (Geffen, Traub, and Stierman, 1978) and others that make it possible to factor out the variables and to determine the relative contributions of each hemisphere to a given task (Moscovitch, 1973; Berlucchi, 1974; Zaidel, personal communication).

One such technique looks at how RT differences between the left and right sensory fields vary with the responding hand in a task that requires a yes-no decision to be signaled by a button press. A consistent sensory-field advantage that is maintained regardless of response hand indicates that the task is functionally localized to a single hemisphere, whereas an interaction of responding hand with sensory field indicates that both hemispheres contribute to performance. By this type of analysis, experiments have shown that tasks requiring phonological decisions are functionally localized to the left hemisphere, a finding consistent with the clinical literature (for reviews see Moscovitch, 1976, 1981). Similarly, some visual pattern-recognition tasks, but by no means all (for example, face recognition) are functionally localized to the right hemisphere (for reviews see Berlucchi, 1974; Moscovitch, 1979; Sergent and Bindra, 1981; Bradshaw and Nettlelon, 1981; Morais, 1982). Although the neurological literature indicates that damage to either hemisphere may impair face recognition (Benton, 1980; Hecaen and Albert, 1978) and that damage to both is usually necessary to produce prosopagnosia (Hecaen and Albert, 1978; Meadows, 1974) the results of studies on normal people suggest that for some face-recognition tasks the left hemisphere's contribution is negligible, whatever its underlying capacity might be (Moscovitch, Scullion, and Christie, 1976).

Table 1
Go/No-Go Reaction Time (in msec) to Concrete and Abstract
Words Presented in Either the Left or the Right Visual Field
[Moscovitch, 1981]

	Left hand		Right hand	
	LVF	RVF	LVF	RVF
Concrete	673	643	674	666
Abstract	671	622	709	643

When applied to other questions, such as the right hemisphere's contribution to processing verbal information semantically, the techniques produce mixed results. For
example, the clinical literature suggests that the right hemisphere has a lexicon consisting primarily of concrete words,
represented semantically, but not easily manipulated phonologically, if at all (Levy and Trevarthen, 1977; Zaidel,
1978a, and the chapter in this book). One would, therefore,
expect abstract and function words to produce a consistent
right-field–left-hemisphere advantage and concrete words to
show no advantage or to produce sensory-field RT differences
that would vary with responding hand. Whereas some studies
do report stronger left-hemisphere advantage for abstract
over concrete words, an equal number of studies have failed
to find any differences (for reviews see Moscovitch, 1981,
Searlman, 1977). Our own studies fall into the latter category.
For example, Janet Olds and I attempted to replicate Day's
(1977, 1979) finding that in a lexical decision task, a consistent left-field advantage is found only for abstract words.
As table 1 shows, there was a right-field–left-hemisphere
advantage for both concrete and abstract words. Although
only the overall right-field advantage was statistically significant, the data are not as conclusive as one would like,
since there is a hint that concrete words did produce smaller
perceptual asymmetries than abstract ones.

What these studies suggest is that regardless of the right
hemisphere's proven capacity to process verbal information

semantically, normal people tend to rely primarily on the left hemisphere's superior abilities in this domain. This type of *functional localization* may occur because the left hemisphere inhibits the right with regard to linguistic functions, because the left hemisphere completes the task before the right or because the subject chooses a strategy that is more compatible with left- than with right-hemisphere processes (Moscovitch, 1973, 1976). Whatever the reason, the right hemisphere's inherent abilities are not reflected in normal performance, so that linguistic functions appear to be localized exclusively to the left hemisphere.

In a sense, the clinical literature supports this hypothesis. At the moment there are only two papers, by Lesser (1974) and by Gainotti and coworkers (1981), that show even a mild semantic impairment in comprehending spoken and written words and sentences following right-hemisphere lesions. Significantly, both studies failed to find impaired syntactic or phonological functions in these patients.

Under some circumstances, however, the right hemisphere's linguistic abilities, particularly its semantic ones, may emerge and may influence performance—even in normal people—as, for example, in the occasional observation of right-hemisphere processing of concrete words. Although the nature of these circumstances has yet to be elaborated, a number of possibilities seem promising. One involves occupying the left hemisphere and thereby enabling the right hemisphere's capacities to emerge. This would be consistent with the model illustrated in figure 13, in which the two hemispheres are conceived as separate, but interdependent, information-processing systems (Moscovitch, 1979). When one system is overloaded, the other's contribution to a particular task may, by comparison, become more evident (Hellige and Cox, 1976; Hellige, Cox, and Litvac, 1979; Friedman and Poulson, 1981).

A second possibility is to present pictorial stimuli or to devise other tasks that may naturally engage the superior

Table 2
Mean Classification Scores[a] [Wilkins and Moscovitch, 1978]

| | "Living–man-made" | | "Larger–smaller" | |
	Drawings	Words	Drawings	Words
Left temporal	12.1	12.3	13.1	13.3
Right temporal	14.4	13.6	13.1	11.4
Normal control	14.5	14.4	12.9	12.5

a. Maximum score, 16. Average chance score, 8.

Table 3
Mean Naming Scores[a] [Wilkins and Moscovitch, 1978]

	Without cue	With cue
Left temporal	11.4	11.6
Right temporal	13.3	12.6
Normal control	14.7	13.9

a. Maximum score, 16.

visuospatial processing mechanisms of the right hemisphere. Wilkins and Moscovitch (1978) found that patients with left temporal lobectomy, but not those with right, had difficulty rapidly naming line drawings or classifying line drawings and words as representing something that is living or man-made. They were, however, perfectly normal at classifying the same material by size, even though control subjects and patients with right temporal lobectomy found this task somewhat more difficult (see tables 2 and 3). Presumably, size classification requires analogical visuospatial processes that depend more on right-hemisphere functions than do naming and taxonomic classification. Similar processes are involved in imagery-mediated verbal recall. Although right temporal lobectomy is not as devastating on verbal recall as left temporal lobectomy, the former does lead to a noticeable impairment of performance on tasks that have a strong imagery component. Jones (1976), confirming Patten (1972), reported that imagery mnemonics improve the performance of patients with left temporal lobectomy, but not of those with right temporal lobectomy, in verbal paired associate tasks. The technique is so effective that one patient who was virtually amnesic for verbal material improved to near-normal levels when concrete words and imagery mnemonics were employed (Moscovitch, unreported). In a subsequent study, Jones-Gotman and Milner (1978) and Jones-Gotman (1979) established that an intact right temporal lobe is critical for normal performance on verbal tasks that have an imagery cmponent, such as recalling concrete, but not abstract, words.

The different contributions of both hemispheres to verbal recall are even more noticeable when pictorial stimuli are used. Jaccarino (1975; compare Milner, 1978) found that damage to either the right or left temporal lobe resulted in impaired recall of the names of line drawings that were presented a day earlier. That damage to the right temporal lobe can influence even *immediate* verbal recall was demonstrated by Moscovitch (1976). He presented patients with sixteen randomly ordered drawings of common objects each of which belonged to one of four taxonomic or shape categories (see figure 14). In recalling the names of these drawings, normal subjects usually cluster their responses according to both lexical and shape categories (Frost, 1972). Patients with right temporal lobectomy, however, clustered only by taxonomic category, while patients with left temporal lobectomy clustered primarily by shape but inconsistently by taxonomic category (table 4).

Similar biases in clustering could be produced in normal people by presenting the drawings with a concurrent task that affects the processing capacities of one hemisphere more than the other. In the concurrent nonverbal task, which is presumed to affect right-hemisphere processing, the subject identifies central nonsense figures while encoding a bilaterally presented drawing (see figure 15). In the concurrent verbal task, left-hemisphere processes are engaged by having the subject name a central, vertically presented word. In the

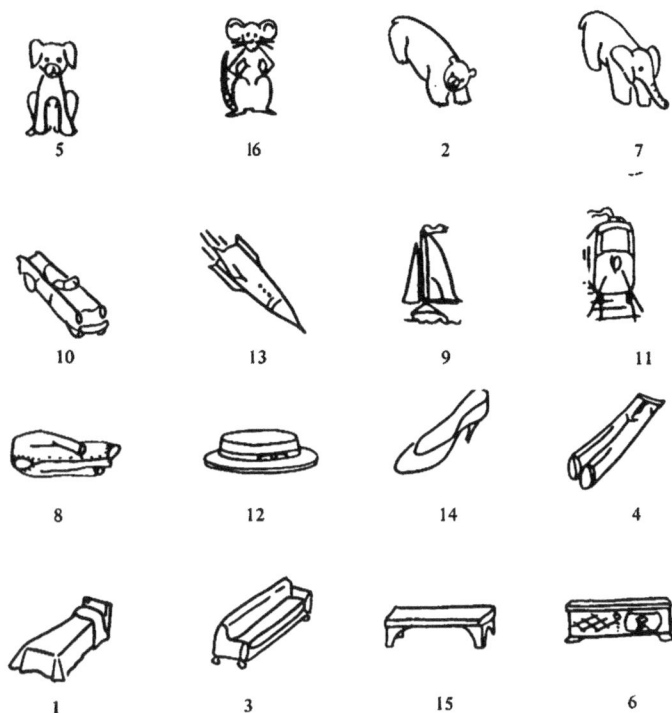

Figure 14.
An example of a set of line drawings presented to the subjects. The number next to each drawing indicated the order of presentation. (I thank Nancy Frost for making these drawings available to me.) (Moscovitch, 1981)

Table 4
Mean Items Recalled and Mean Clustering for Spatial and
Verbal Categories [Moscovitch, 1981]

	Mean items recalled	Spatial ARC[a]	Verbal ARC[a]
Left temporal	8.5	0.27	0.34
Right temporal	10.7	0.07	0.31
Normal control	11.0	0.14	0.36

a. ARC = adjusted ratio for clustering (Roenker, Thompson, and Brown, 1971).

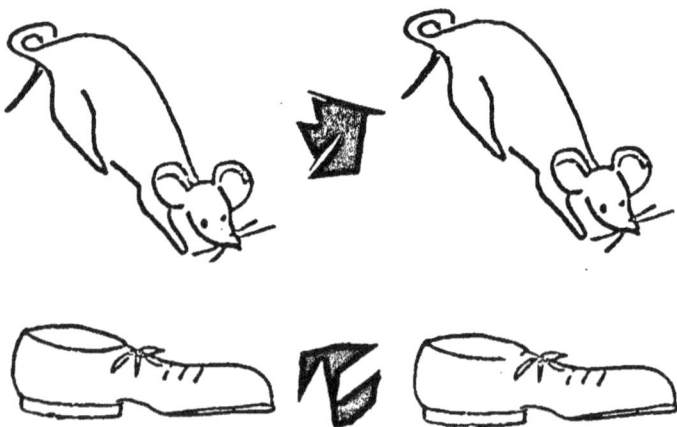

Figure 15.
Example of two line drawings and the accompanying neutral, nonverbal interfering stimuli that were presented tachistoscopically. (Moscovitch, 1981)

Table 5
Mean Items Recalled and Mean Clustering for Spatial and
Verbal Categories [Moscovitch, 1981]

	Mean items recalled	Spatial ARC[a]	Verbal ARC[a]
Nonverbal concurrent	7.2	−0.19	0.39
Verbal concurrent	4.2	0.37	0.04
Control	8.5	0.12	0.20

a. ARC = adjusted ratio for clustering (Roenker, Thompson, and Brown, 1971).

control condition, the center is left blank. As table 5 shows, taxonomic clustering is predominant in the nonverbal concurrent condition, and spatial clustering in the verbal concurrent condition. The possibility of right-hemisphere involvement in dual coding is discussed at length by Paivio and te Linde (1982).

These results are consistent with our hypothesis that beyond the early stage of processing each hemisphere encodes the identical information in a manner commensurate with its abilities. On verbal tasks, however, special techniques are required to free the right hemisphere from the dominance of the left and to reveal its contribution to normal performance.

Apart from memory, the domain in which the right hemisphere's contributions to verbal performance are most evident is not that of traditional linguistics, such as phonology, syntax, and semantics, but rather the paralinguistic aspects of language, such as intonation, emotional tone, context, inference, and connotation—in short, those aspects of language that may be included as part of pragmatics or the discourse function of language (Bates, 1976). Patients with right-hemisphere lesions react inappropriately to humorous material (Gardner et al., 1975; Wapner, Hamby, and Gardner, in press), interpret metaphors incorrectly (Winner and Gardner, 1977), have a poor appreciation of antonymic contrasts (Gardner et al., 1978) and the connotative aspects of pictures (Gardner and Denes, 1973), and have difficulty producing and perceiving the correct emotional tone of linguistic utterances (Heilman, Scholes, and Watson, 1975; Ross and Mesulam, 1979). These observations are consistent with results of laterality studies in normal people (see, for example, Blumstein and Cooper, 1974; Haggard and Parkinson, 1971; Safer and Leventhal, 1977; Zurif, 1974). Patients with right-hemisphere damage seem to have no difficulty comprehending individual sentences; but they do have difficulty relating a sentence to a larger context, understanding its emotional connotation, and drawing the proper inferences from it (Wapner et al., in press). Without the right hemisphere, communication, in its broadest sense, seems not to proceed normally.

Despite possessing some syntactic and considerable lexical-semantic competence, the right hemisphere seems to contribute little to normal linguistic performance in these domains. In order to convey and apprehend the literal straightforward linguistic truth, the left hemisphere seems sufficient under most circumstances. If the truth is to be embellished with vocal nuances, appropriate turns of phrase and bons mots, in short, if the domain of language is to be expanded to include all those functions that ordinarily enter into normal discourse, then the right hemisphere's contribution, though elusive, may yet turn out to be as significant as some recent research suggests.

On Multiple Representations of the Lexicon in the Brain— The Case of Two Hemispheres

E. Zaidel

In 1933 Shepherd Ivory Franz, the first chairman of the Psychology Department at UCLA, former president of the American Psychological Association (1920), and neuropsychologist extraordinaire, published three papers in which he reported and interpreted a set of experiments on hemispheric specialization in normal subjects (Franz and Davis, 1933; Franz and Kilduff, 1933; Franz, 1933). Using a surprisingly modern experimental design for tachistoscopic presentations, Franz obtained a left visual half-field advantage (LVFA) for reading single four-letter words, split 10 degrees apart across the fixation. He also observed a right visual half-field advantage (RVFA) for identifying bilateral nonsense geometric shapes. And he found smaller, but not reversed, laterality effects in left-handers than in right-handers. Partly because of these unexpected results, this at a time when the left cerebral hemisphere (LH) was believed to be dominant for language and other higher functions alike, and when left-handers were believed to have a dominant right cerebral hemisphere (RH), mirror-image fashion, Franz concluded that the concept of cerebral dominance is psychological rather than biological, in the sense that it is sensitive to task parameters that can shift control from one hemisphere to the other.

Franz's anomalous reading results can most probably be attributed to reading scanning habits powerfully induced by the task, Read a word split apart, whose first half occurs in the peripheral LVF. And almost twenty years later, when Mishkin and Forgays (1952) initiated their own studies of reading in the two visual half-fields, they in turn rejected a hemispheric interpretation of the observed RVFA for English words in favor of an explanation in terms of reading scanning habit. What was missing in both the UCLA and McGill experiments was a compelling rationale for interpreting the observed laterality effects as evidence of hemispheric specialization. Such a rationale was provided in a particularly dramatic form in 1960 by the human split-brain syndrome, both in its natural variety studied by Geschwind and Kaplan (1962) and in its surgical variety in the experiments initiated by Sperry, Gazzaniga, and Bogen at Caltech. The pioneering studies of Vogel and Bogen's commissurotomy patients demonstrated that each disconnected hemisphere constitutes a fairly complete cognitive system, with its own perceptions, memories, problem-solving strategies, language, even personality, and "consciousness" (Sperry, Gazzaniga, and Bogen, 1969). The split brain experiments offer an operational definition for the concept "degree of hemispheric specialization" and provide several possible models for interpreting laterality effects in normal subjects (Zaidel, 1982b).

A common interpretation of the split-brain data is that each hemisphere is specialized for a particular cognitive style that characterizes both its nonlinguistic and its linguistic behavior. The LH may be specialized for abstract algorithmic or combinatoric analysis; the RH may be specialized for template matching of patterns formed from direct experience. In the following comments I would like to use the example of a receptive lexicon to illustrate the idea of multiple representations of cognitive structures in the brain. The LH lexicon corresponds to our common linguistic intuitions, but the RH lexicon is organized differently and seems adapted to the cognitive specialization of that hemisphere. Can these observations be generalized to the normal brain? In my concluding comments I shall suggest that a strong generalization may well be justified.

Let me now review briefly some of the results on the structure of the lexicon in the disconnected RH. Consider the auditory, orthographic, and semantic (pictorial) representations of a reference word. The disconnected LH is facile in translating across all three representations. What about the RH? To find out, we have used a contact-lens technique that makes it possible for one hemisphere at a time to scan freely a complex visual stimulus. In the case of printed words or pictures, vision is simply restricted either to the LVF or RVF, allowing either the RH or LH, respectively, to scan the stimuli. In the case of spoken words, a multiple choice array of four or five pictures is lateralized to one VF. The auditory stimulus reaches both hemispheres, but only one hemisphere sees the multiple choices and can make the association of the correct picture with the spoken word.

By using the Peabody Picture Vocabulary Test it was found that the two tested disconnected RHs had a surprisingly rich auditory vocabulary ranging from the equivalent of a 12- to an 18-year-old normal child (figure 16). Although both disconnected hemispheres showed the same dependence on word frequency as the corresponding LHs with a similar drop-off for low-frequency words, the RH vocabulary was consistently smaller and seemed to be more connotative than denotative. Thus, there seem to exist at least two separate auditory lexicons in the split brain, one in each hemisphere.

The auditory RH lexicon can be differentiated from the LH lexicon also in its grammatical function. Using a test developed as part of a much larger battery for assessing semantic and syntactic aspects of auditory language comprehension by Susie Curtiss and Jenny Yamada at UCLA, we found that in the case of pluralization the RH is more likely to include in its repertoire those grammatical distinctions that can be signaled lexically, such as the auxiliary "is"

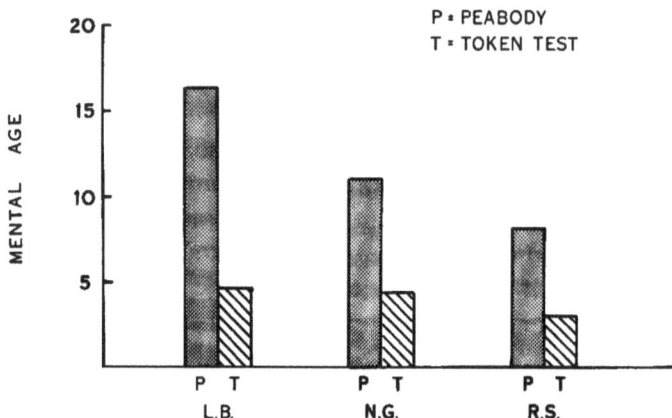

Figure 16.
Equivalent mental ages of commissurotomy patients L.B. and
N.G. and of left, dominant hemispherectomy patient R.S. on the
Peabody and Ammon Picture Vocabulary Tests (comprehension
of spoken words) and on the Token Test (comprehension of spo-
ken phrases). (Zaidel)

versus "are" (the fish is eating/the fish are eating), than those
signaled morphologically, such as the third-person-singular
inflection "s"(the fish eats/the fish eat) (figures 17, 18). Also,
RH comprehension seems to vary as a function of part of
speech (figure 19).

I do not think that poor short-term verbal memory or
weak auditory discrimination completely accounts for the
syntactic deficit of the RH. First, auditory discrimination in
the RH is not all that poor (Zaidel, 1978a). Second, its short-
term verbal memory is usually sufficient for two to three
words. Finally, the syntactic effects occur at both the sentential and lexical level (Zaidel, 1978b). Again, I think the
evidence points to a RH auditory lexicon that is organized
differently and hence is also represented separately from the
auditory lexicon of the LH. This conclusion would be supported even if the grammatical deficit of the RH could be

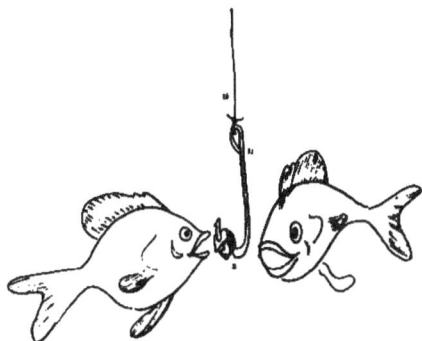

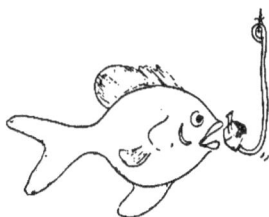

Figure 17.
An item from Curtiss and Yamada's test of pluralization: "The
fish eats/"The fish eat" (inflections) or "The fish is eating"/"The
fish are eating" (auxiliaries). (Zaidel)

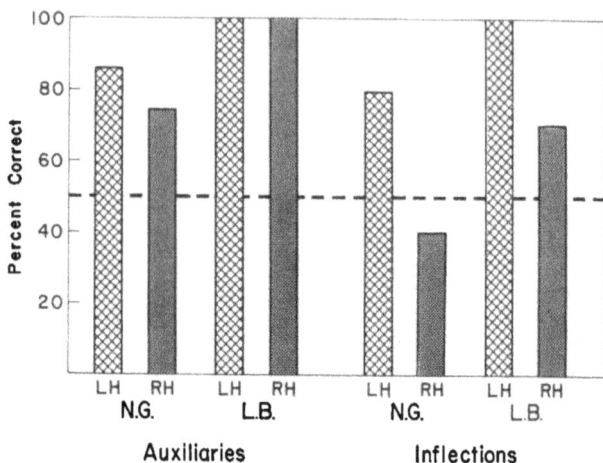

Figure 18.
Unilateral scores of the left hemispheres (LH) and right hemispheres (RH) of commissurotomy patients N.G. and L.B. on the
auxiliaries and inflections versions of Curtiss and Yamada's test
for comprehension of pluralization. (Zaidel)

accounted for completely in terms of a weak auditory discrimination or a poor short-term verbal memory. Such
weaknesses must mean that the RH uses alternative strategies
for its extensive lexical decoding. Both the weaknesses and
the alternative strategies amount to a different organization
and thus a separate cortical representation.

Consider next the reading vocabulary of the RH. Using
a reading version of the Peabody Picture Vocabulary Test
and a separate spelling test, we obtained similar age scores
that were consistently lower than those obtained for the auditory vocabulary (about 10 years of age for patient L.B.'s
RH, about 7 years for patient N.G.'s RH.) Moreover, the
visual vocabulary seemed to constitute a proper subset of
the auditory vocabulary; we never observed cases where the
RH could read a word that it could not understand when
spoken. In fact, the RH cannot translate orthography into

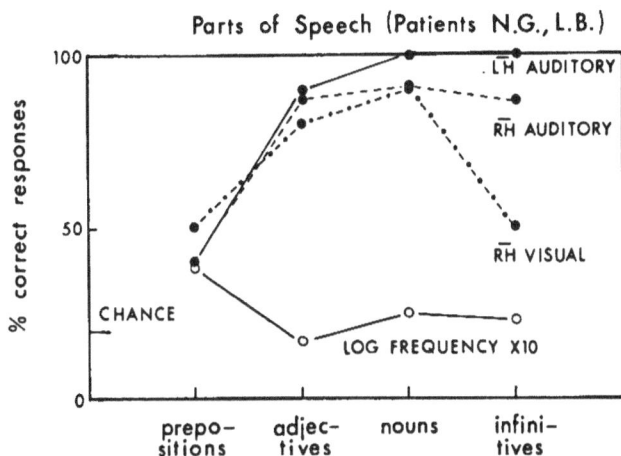

Figure 19.
Mean unilateral right-hemisphere scores on reading and auditory comprehension tests using the same words, as a function of part of speech. Mean log frequency × 10 (per million—Thorndike and Lorge) for each word category is indicated for comparison. (Zaidel)

sound. This was demonstrated directly by its inability to match reliably meaningful or nonsense rhyming words (figure 20). The RH could not match the same meaningful rhyming words that it could read quite well in the sense of matching them with their pictorial referents or in the sense of matching the spoken name with its correct spelling. In the case of nonsense words, the RHs could match them neither for rhyming nor with the spoken names. It would seem to follow that the RH has never acquired grapheme-to-phoneme correspondence rules and therefore reads without intermediate phonetic recoding.

This means again that the RH lexicon is organized quite differently from that of the LH, where transformations from any lexical representation to another are available once phonetic reading has been acquired. Further, the fact that the

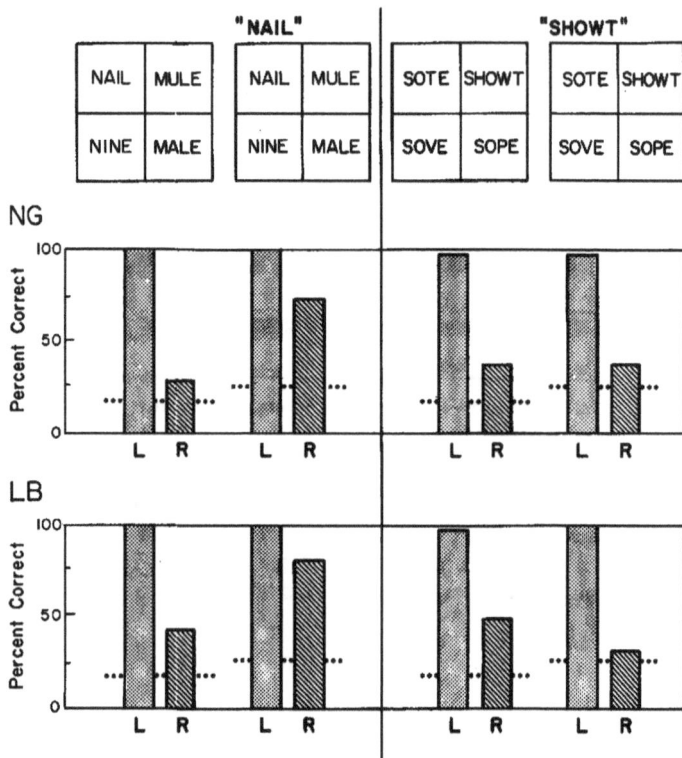

Figure 20.
Scores of the left (L) and right (R) hemispheres of patients N.G. and L.B. on two tests of rhyming, one for meaningful words and the other for nonsense words, and their controls. The rhyming tests require pointing to the two rhyming words in stimulus quartets. The control tests require pointing to the word spoken by the examiner. The rhyming tests have several parts, hence the variable chance levels denoted by a dotted line. (Zaidel)

RH can match a spoken word with its spelling in the case of meaningful, but not nonsense, words would suggest that the RH does have some ability to evoke the visual representation of a heard word, but that this ability is a learned association through experience and therefore limited to previously encountered real words, rather than constituting phoneme-grapheme translation rules, which would apply equally well to real and nonsense words.

Other clues to the unique organization of the RH lexicon come from multiple-choice reading tests where the foils are carefully selected to provide visual, auditory, and semantic confusions with the target stimulus. In this paradigm, the RHs make more semantic than either auditory or visual errors in reading, and these errors tend to be syntagmatic rather than paradigmatic (Zaidel, 1982a).

Furthermore, the access routes available "to and from" the RH lexicon may be selectively limited. For example, the RH seems rarely able to execute written commands even though it can match a spoken or a written command with its pictorial representation. This seems unrelated to apraxia; these RHs can imitate complex gestures and can even initiate them in the proper nonlinguistic context (D. Zaidel and Sperry, 1977).

Given the rich auditory lexicon of the RHs, the next question is, How well can they understand longer spoken phrases? The answer is, Not very well. One example of this is the contrast between the high mental-age equivalents of RH scores on the picture vocabulary tests and their surprisingly low-age scores on the Token Test (figure 16). Rather like aphasic patients, the RHs find it very difficult to decode nonredundant context-free phrases like "Point to the large green square and the small yellow circle." Possibly, the RHs, as well as many receptive and expressive aphasics, suffer from a limited short-term verbal memory, since they do not have access to a constructive phonological rehearsal buffer.

Such a rehearsal buffer could be used to store one part of the auditory message while decoding another.

It seems possible that the RH should be able to read longer sentences than it can understand aurally. The auditory message is fleeting, whereas the visual sentence is continuously present throughout the decoding process, however long it lasts. This turns out not to be the case. The RH has the same falloff curve as a function of length, for both auditory and printed phrases, with the visual material yielding constantly worse performance. A likely explanation is that the internal representation of the visual input is not iconic and again requires phonological encoding for rehearsal and maintenance in short-term memory. Certainly, to argue that the RH reads without phonetic recoding is not to argue that it reads words as fixed visual templates or gestalts. After all, the RH can read across different typefaces, cases, sizes, and handwriting styles.

An attractive interpretation of RH lexical capacity is due to Studdert-Kennedy and Shankweiler and argues that RH competence is restricted to auditory, without phonetic, analysis (Studdert-Kennedy and Shankweiler, 1970). This would be consistent with the absence of speech in the RH. But the RH occasionally appears to have a rudimentary constructive phonological capacity in the sense of matching two pictures with homonymous or rhyming names. More disturbingly, the RH has "duplex perception" in the sense of Liberman, Isenberg, and Rakerd (1981). When normal subjects are presented with a dichotic pair consisting of the common "base" (first two formants and third formant without its transition— see figure 1) of the synthetic words *rock/lock* channeled to one ear, and of the third formant transition identifying one of the words (say, *rock*) channeled to the other ear, there occurs a "duplex percept," with the fused word (*rock*) heard in one ear, and a chirp, associated with the isolated third formant transition, heard in the other ear. Liberman argues cogently for the chirp perception as an auditory or acoustic event, but for the fused word percept as a phonetic event. Studdert-Kennedy and Shankweiler's interpretation would then suggest that the fused percept should only occur in the LH. However, a pilot experiment with David Isenberg disclosed duplex perception in either ear of several split-brain patients. Unilateral responses were obtained by restricting a visual probe consisting of the picture of either a lock, a rock, or a frog to one visual half-field following the dichotic pair and asking the subject to point to "yes" or "no" with the hand ipsilateral to the stimulated half-field.

Rather than interpret these findings (provided they are supported by further experiments) as suggesting that the RH can analyze acoustic events phonetically, I would suggest instead that the fusion of the two ear signals occurs at a subcortical level and does not require RH phonetic processing. Certainly, the paradigm does not create ipsilateral suppression and so allows access of both ears to both hemispheres.

The ultimate question is whether the normal RH has functional receptive language that respects the limits found in the laboratory for the disconnected RH. We started answering this by selecting a simple linguistic task, that is, lexical decision, that seems to tap a relatively early and automatic stage in reading, yet is sensitive to lexical semantics through facilitation. Three tasks were used. In the first, visual priming task, a briefly lateralized (100-millisecond) word is flashed randomly either to the left or to the right of fixation. This is called the "prime," and the subject is instructed to ignore it. After a 500-millisecond delay, another lateralized (50-millisecond) character string is flashed either to the same or the opposite half-field. This is called the "target," and the subject is instructed to show by a button press whether this is a real English word or not. The nonwords are all orthographically legal strings, and for this experiment they were formed by replacing one letter in a real word. For half of the target words, the prime is semantically related to the

LB   VISUAL   PRIMING

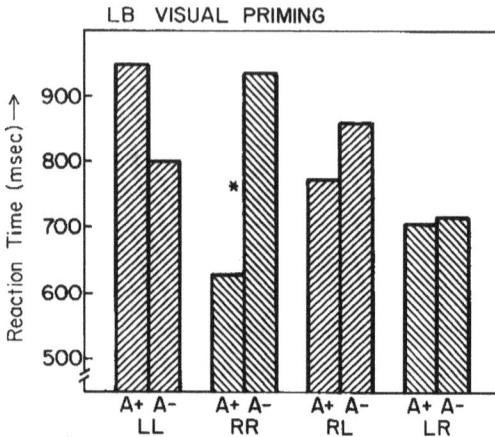

Figure 21.
Performance of commissurotomy patient L.B. on the lexical decision and visual priming task. A−, A+ denote responses to targets with unassociated and associated primes, respectively. LL = left visual half-field (LVF) primes and LVF targets; LR = LVF primes and RVF targets, and so on. * = statistically significant difference between A+ and A− ($P < 0.05$).

target ("associated" or A+ condition). Reaction-time studies in normal subjects show faster responses to words than to nonwords, and faster responses to associated than unassociated pairs ("facilitation"). In the second, auditory priming task, the lateralized visual primes were replaced by spoken ones. In the third, only targets, with no primes, were presented.

The visual priming task administered to five commissurotomy patients showed bilateral competence for lexical decision, with more accurate but not faster LH performance. Only one patient, L.B., showed semantic facilitation, and only in the LH (figure 21). The auditory priming task, on the other hand, in addition to showing bilateral lexical decision also yielded bilateral facilitation with no consistent hemispheric superiorities (figure 22). As can be expected, the

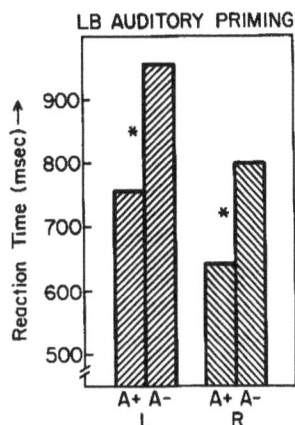

Figure 22.
Performance of patient L.B. on the lexical decision and auditory priming task. L = LVF targets; R = RVF targets. (Zaidel)

"targets only" task yielded bilateral lexical decision, but it also showed significant though mixed hemispheric superiorities. Thus both hemispheres have the capacity for lexical decision, and the disconnected RHs had auditory but not visual facilitation. Previous findings of interhemispheric noncallosal facilitation (Zaidel, 1982a) were not confirmed when subjected to further controls.

The lexical decision and semantic facilitation task was designed and administered to normal subjects by Allen Radant, an honors psychology undergraduate at UCLA. Extensions of the test showed bilateral hemispheric competence for lexical decision and visual semantic facilitation in normal subjects. The evidence that each normal hemisphere performed the task to a definite extent independently of the other comes from comparison between performance on the visual priming task and that on the targets alone. Considering only trials where primes and targets reached the same hemisphere, the difference between the two tasks interacted significantly with hemisphere of presentation (Zaidel, 1982b).

The implication of the split-brain and normal study together is that the disconnected RH actually underestimates the contribution of the normal RH to reading. The normal LH seems to support RH involvement in reading so that "two hemispheres are better than one" even for such a linguistic task.

There remains the issue of actual RH contribution to the normal auditory comprehension or reading process. We have observed three hemispherectomy patients, one dominant and two nondominant, where the surgeries were performed for postinfantile malignancies, and found them to have dramatically varying degrees of reading competence. These patients may provide hints on development and use of reading in the RH. Patient R.S. had complete dominant hemispherectomy for a glioma at age 10 with symptoms at age 7. She remained nonfluently aphasic with better comprehension than speech and no reading. Patient D.W., who had been left-handed but showed LH speech on amytal testing, lost his RH at age 7 due to encephalitis, with first symptoms at age 6. He remains severely dyslexic, dysgraphic, and dyscalculic. He has visuospatial deficits; his speech and comprehension are good; and his writing is poor though phonetic. Finally, patient G.E. had right, nondominant hemispherectomy for a tumor at age 30 and retained her language, including good reading, though not her visuospatial and musical abilities. Together these cases suggest that the RH may play a special role in reading acquisition. Supporting evidence comes from studies of normal children who are learning how to read (see, for example, Silverberg et al., 1980; Bakker and Moerland, 1981).

A complementary hypothesis would argue that the RH is also important for speed-reading, where quick orientation to recurring visual patterns is important. Little supporting data for this hypothesis are available at the present time. But this may be due to the failure to use sensitive clinical tests that will pick up subtle deficits in reading, such as quick paragraph perusal, following right-hemisphere damage. The recent trend has been toward closing the gap between the hemisphere-damaged, commissurotomy, and normal data concerning language representation in the brain. No single paradigm is sufficient, and convergent evidence seems our best goal.

How does the split-brain work bear on the problem of language autonomy? I think that the disconnection syndrome clarifies and highlights some of the issues in a particularly dramatic way, but that its ultimate interpretation remains ambiguous. Disconnection may be said to outline the limits of hemispheric competence, but it may still describe potential rather than actual normal conditions. There is no doubt that the disconnected LH is specialized for language and for some related perceptual/cognitive oprations. Speech is most lateralized to the left, and phonetic analysis and syntax seem to be the paradigmatic LH language functions. The RH, on the other hand, can handle single lexical items and seems to have a rich conceptual/semantic system and to be capable of superior handling of certain pragmatic and extralinguistic aspects of communication. For example, the RH may play a particularly important role in nonverbal communication, such as the interpretation of the affective-social significance of facial expressions and body movements (Benowitz et al., 1982). On the nonlinguistic side, the RH may be especially important for certain visuospatial tasks, such as experience-reinforced template matching and gestalt completion, whereas the LH may be better at feature extraction and figure-ground separation as in embedded-figure tasks (field independence). Thus the two cerebral hemispheres are specialized for related linguistic as well as related nonlinguistic cognitive operations, and the relation between these two specializations remains unclear.

The difficulties are, first, that there is no a priori agreement on what constitutes the core of language, especially vis-à-vis the more general communicative situation and the particular sensorimotor vehicles used to carry the interaction. Second, it is difficult to determine the teleological status of linguistic versus other cognitive abilities in the LH. Is language specialization in the LH the consequence of a more general and earlier LH specialization for motor control? Or are the cognitive superiorities of the LH consequences of sharing the apparatus evolved for and shaped by language use? If we accept the theoretical linguistic (Chomskian) characterization of language and ask for validation of its autonomy by cortical separability, then the split-brain data offer at best moderate support. But the alternative approach is equally justified: Look at what the LH is specialized for and call that the essential core of language. Then neurological separability is a tautology. Furthermore, there is an everyday, commonsense view of language as a vehicle for commmunication. It would seem that both hemispheres are used for total communication in that sense, and that in the resulting interactions it is difficult to separate strictly linguistic from cognitive factors.

Right-hemisphere (RH) involvement in language processing can perhaps be summarized by saying that it can contribute to semantic and pragmatic, and thus also paralinguistic, processes. The LH, on the other hand, may be specialized for phonology and syntax, both in the concrete sense of phonetic speech analysis and complex syntactic transformations and in the more abstract sense of representing an algorithmic combinatorial structure modeled by a generative grammar. RH competence in handling lexical items is then an example of its more general capacity for abstraction and labeling and of its specific capacity for processing extralinguistic significance or meaning in communication, as in pictures (D. Zaidel, 1981), facial affect and body postures (Benowitz et al., 1982) and prosody (Ross, 1981). In particular, the RH may be important in the connotative interpretation of lexical items, the thematic interpretation of discourse, the analysis of suprasegmental features, and the interpretation of paralinguistic elements during communication.

All this is quite consistent with Moscovitch's interpretation. Two sorts of validation are required. First, we should be able to observe some linguistic deficits following some right-hemisphere lesions. The classical failure to find such deficits can, at least partly, be attributed to a failure to look for them. Indeed the roles of the RH in theme perception, discourse analysis, and prosody have all been inferred from recent brain-damage studies. With appropriately subtle tests we should similarly be able to verify impaired connotative appreciation of lexical items, and so on. In the specific case of reading we already have very preliminary brain-damage evidence that the RH is necessary for reading acquisition, though not for maintaining basic reading once acquired. Finally, a special role for the RH in quick efficient reading may be demonstrated by proper tests that are rarely performed in the clinic.

Another aspect of the same validation criterion would require us to show that the RH can support language processing following aphasia due to LH damage to an extent consistent with RH competence, as demonstrated in commissurotomy studies. Now that the possibility has been explicitly stated, neurological evidence in its support is becoming frequent (see, for example, Cummings et al., 1979). Still, one should expect a considerable amount of individual variation in RH language competence. Also, pathological inhibition of healthy RH cortex by diseased LH tissue may occur in certain lesions. Such inhibition could perhaps be demonstrated experimentally by removing it with certain psychological manipulations, such as concurrent loading in dual task paradigms.

The second sort of validation of RH language is a demonstration of it in the normal brain. All those half-field tachistoscopic laterality effects for reading in normal subjects that satisfy the "direct-access" interpretation (each hemisphere processes its own input for better or worse; Zaidel, 1982b) support the conclusion of some language role for the normal RH. Certainly the occurrence of an RVFA on some linguistic hemifield tachistoscopic task does not mean that the normal RH is not involved. My own data suggest that such a role is tapped by lexical decision. I believe that RH contribution to normal language processing is unique and strengthens LH processing of the task.

Comments: N. Geschwind

Moscovitch notes that the lack of evidence for impaired semantic comprehension and nonphonetic reading comprehension after right-hemisphere damage is disturbing in view of reports that the right hemisphere may support these activities after left-sided damage. Zaidel argues that commissurotomy studies support the presence of many linguistic capacities in the right hemisphere and that the lack of clinical evidence may only indicate a failure of adequate testing.

Perhaps Zaidel is correct. However, a possible alternative explanation should be considered. First, an assumption implicitly accepted by investigators of commissurotomies is that the distribution of functions after surgical separation of the hemispheres reflects that found in the brains of most normal adults. Yet, with only one exception, all the split-brain patients have had long-standing epilepsy, beginning early and based on either prenatal or early-childhood brain disorder. Since it is well-known that both prenatal and postnatal disorders alter brain organization (almost certainly in different ways) and that long-standing epilepsy itself may lead to reorganization, the commissurotomy cases, as well as the hemispherectomies, may reflect in some (perhaps most) cases the effects of postlesion changes in the nervous system of the kind discussed by Ojemann in part II of this book: (1) The redundant capacities of the right hemisphere may be present but suppressed in the normal and only released as a result of lesion; (2) alternatively (and perhaps more likely), when the normal function of the right hemisphere is destroyed, other systems not normally involved in language compensate, producing a partial recovery that may be mistakenly construed as an uninvolved residue of normal function. Many of the characteristics of deep dyslexia depend, in my view, on such a mechanism. These explanations may not be correct, but they should be considered.

Comments

The study of hemispheric specialization seems to invite grand dichotomies: temporal-spatial, analytic-holistic, intellectual-emotional. But, presumably, a behavioral mode does not evolve without a behavior to support, and our task begins, rather than ends, with such descriptive oppositions (Studdert-Kennedy, 1981a). Once they are established, we must subvert them by tracing their origins and adaptive functions.

What, for example, are we to make of the (somewhat tenuous) abstract-concrete opposition discussed by Moscovitch? How, if it is valid, might it arise? An attractive suggestion, offered during discussion, was that an apparent left-hemisphere superiority in the processing of abstract words might reflect the kind of syntactically enriched lexicon that Caplan has described in this part. Abstract words, such as *fact, hope, hatred*, and so on, frequently govern, or at least imply, complements (*the fact that . . . , her hope of . . . , his hatred of . . .*). Thus we might trace the left hemisphere's possible predilection for abstract words to its syntactic skill.

But what are we to make of its syntactic skill? The evidence from both normal subjects and split-brain patients, reviewed earlier, is consistent with a view of the left hemisphere as the locus of specialized modules for the two levels of structure, phonology and syntax, that seem to distinguish language from other systems of communication. Moreover, the right hemisphere seems to complement the left, with its pragmatic and paralinguistic capacities. How did this dissociation arise? By default? By adaptive distribution of neurologically incompatible functions (Semmes, 1968; Levy, 1974)? From prior specializations for perceptuomotor control (Kimura, 1979)?

At least two directions of research hold out some promise of our penetrating more deeply into the nature of these linguistic functions. One is the general direction of continued neuroanatomical study, as argued by Geschwind in part II. Despite skepticism concerning the fit of form to function — a skepticism often justified analogically by noting the diversity of software programs that can be executed by computer hardware — much can be learned from the study of structure. As Geschwind remarks, our understanding of color vision has been built not only on behavioral studies but also on biochemical knowledge. There is no reason to believe that the same will not ultimately be true of our understanding of language.

A second promising direction is through the study of sign language. The discovery that American Sign Language (ASL) has a dual pattern of formational structure and syntax, analogous to that of spoken language, may permit us to dissociate language from its modality of expression. No other animal, so far as we know, has developed two functionally equivalent, *primary* modes of communication, exploiting different sensorimotor systems. (Reading, writing, and the various tactile systems, such as Braille, are, of course, *secondary* modes, contingent on the discovery of writing systems to represent spoken language.) Moreover, we may doubt whether humans could have developed any alternative primary system other than that of oromanual sign language. Only the hand, face, and vocal apparatus have the delicacy and precision of motor control necessary for rapid, informationally dense sequences of gesture fitted to the demands of memory and linguistic communication (see the chapter by Bellugi in part IV).

Thus systematic comparison of the development and aphasic breakdown of language, in native speakers and signers, may permit us to learn how cerebral organization is shaped by language modality. Neville (1975, 1980; Neville, Kutas, and Schmidt, 1982) has already demonstrated different patterns of event-related potentials in the recognition of line drawings, presented to left and right visual fields, for normal children, congenitally deaf children who did not use ASL, and congenitally deaf children who did use ASL. The nonsigning deaf children showed no evidence of hemispheric asymmetry, while the signing deaf children displayed asymmetries opposite in direction to those of the hearing children. Evidently (and not unexpectedly) hemispheric specialization may be a consequence, no less than a condition, of language learning.

Naming Disorders   D. F. Benson

Anomia is the most common aphasic disorder, being present in almost every aphasic patient and also occurring in some common nonaphasic disorders. Not all anomias are the same, and by using clinical observations, a number of phenomenologically different types of anomia can be demonstrated.

1. *Word-production anomia*

a. *Articulatory initiation* Some aphasic patients cannot name an object (for example, comb), but a cue, the initial consonant or an open-ended sentence, often produces the correct name. This is seen most typically in Broca's aphasia.

b. *Paraphasic* Some aphasics produce an answer to naming requests with the correct number of syllables, but substitute one or more phonemes, producing a neologistic response. Most often this occurs in conduction aphasia.

2. *Word-selection anomia* In "pure" anomia the subject cannot produce the name of an object, but recognizes the name and can give a correct description of the use of the object. The most pure anomia is found when there is damage to area 37 of inferotemporal cortex.

3. *Semantic anomia* In anomia of this type, words appear to lose their semantic value; though a subject may repeat the word correctly, the object cannot be named, and when the name is offered, the object cannot be selected. This dis-

order is usually seen when there is injury to the angular gyrus.

4. *Category-specific anomia*   This is a disconnection syndrome in which the subject has notable naming disabiity in only a single category (for example, colors, body parts). The pathology is located in various parts of the posterior hemispheres, separating the angular gyrus from selected sensory areas.

5. *Modality-specific anomia*   This also is a disconnection syndrome; for instance, a subject cannot identify an object by one sensory modality (for example, sight), but names it by others (hearing or touch). Visual agnosia is one example of such an anomia.

6. *Disconnection anomia*   Following section of the corpus callosum, the isolated right hemisphere cannot name objects palpated in the left hand.

7. *Anomia of dementia*   Both Alzheimer's disease and Pick's disease produce serious naming problems that are somewhat different from any of the above (and from each other).

8. *Nonaphasic misnaming*   This disturbance, a substitution of one object name for another, is seen most clearly in acute confusional states.

9. *Psychogenic anomia*   A rare disorder.

   To illustrate the complexity and extent of the brain areas involved in the apparently simple act of naming a presented object, consider the following highly simplified account of how information might travel in the central nervous system. The process is described as a sequence for expository reasons, but, of course, several stages might develop concurrently, in parallel. First, some sort of "picture" of an object, bioelectrochemical in form, travels from the visual input system to the cortex for processing in area 17, the primary visual area. Area 17 has connections to areas 18 and 19, the secondary or visual association areas. From here runs a number of long cortical-cortical connections, including a transcallosal pathway connecting visual association areas of the two hemispheres, an occipital-frontal connection, and an infero-temporal connection. For making a verbal response, the most crucial connection is probably to the angular gyrus, a tertiary association area allowing cross-modal associations. From the angular gyrus connection to area 37 in the temporal lobe seems to be necessary, since damage to area 37 produces loss of naming without loss of recognition of the object or its name. From area 37 information must presumably be projected forward to the motor area for organization of a response, and finally to the brain stem for articulation of the name of the pictured object.

This minimal outline describes only those parts of the cerebrum that seem to be essential for the most efficient production of the name of a single object. While this complex activity is occurring, many other associations with the pictured object are probably also being activated, and some of these may be able to drive alternative pathways for name production. It is obvious that the act of naming demands intactness of a great deal of the brain and can be affected by abnormalities over a wide area. It is also obvious that any research on naming that treats it as a holistic, unitary, linguistic function is naive and likely to be worthless. Moreover, just as diverse functions, processes, and neuroanatomical areas are involved in naming (and are reflected in the diversity of naming problems), so, we may presume, are there diverse underpinnings to other language functions. Realistic divisions of these functions must be established and correlated with neuroanatomy for meaningful research in psycholinguistics.

Word Retrieval for Production   H. Goodglass

The most regularly used experimental task in the study of word retrieval, naming pictured objects, is somewhat artificial, but this does not detract from its value as a probe to reveal how aphasia affects the naming functions. We shall consider two major issues. First, are there stages to naming? One might propose a sequence such as (1) arousal of concept or intention, (2) phonological access, (3) motor execution. It is desirable to support such hypotheses with data from the behavior of groups of patients. Second, we would like to know both the relation between acts of lexical intake and lexical output and also the central representation of the knowledge of a word. We have already noted that there are dissociations between input and output performance for some categories of words, so that even if there is a central representation, it may not always be used.

Problems in word retrieval extend beyond the realm of aphasia—for example, everyday failures to recall proper nouns, such as peoples' names, and the benign naming difficulties of middle-age onset; we are not here considering oral reading or disorders of access to writing names.

One of the intriguing questions about naming is whether a name is a "fact" about the concept to which it refers—for example, like the fact that the United States has fifty states—for which memory can be impaired as for any other fact. If you cannot recall that a particular man is named "John," this does not generally mean that you have forgotten the lexical term "John" as an English word. In contrast, aphasia appears to damage the storage and/or retrieval of the lexical element itself; but in addition it may share with other forms of name-retrieval difficulty the memory link between word and referent. Moreover, nonlinguistic factors, such as rigidity of approach or defects of the search mechanism, can impair naming in those instances where the immediate association fails and a more active word search takes over.

Let us consider naming in terms of a hypothetical flow diagram. There may first be a *supramodal concept*, which can be tapped by any sensory input mode. There seems to be a continuum of levels of arousal of this concept. The intention to say may or may not be enough to trigger naming.

We can ask whether the path from sensory input to naming is mediated by a central concept or whether there is a set of autonomous paths from each sense to the name. Modality-specific anomias do exist—do they always depend on the interruption of input from the sensory system at a point that should be considered to lie outside the language area?

In a study of this question, patients were asked to name 48 objects by looking at a picture of each. Sixteen of them were objects that a normal person would be able to identify also by smell (for example, chocolate, gasoline), 16 of them would be identifiable also by touch (for example, a spoon, scissors), and the remaining 16 also by the sound of action upon them (for example, a bell, a typewriter). Twenty-four aphasics, 12 nonaphasic brain-damaged patients, and 12 normal controls were asked to name each of the 48 objects in response both to its picture and to a presentation in its other input modality. All three groups displayed the same general relation between naming response latencies in pictured and nonpictured conditions. One word-deaf patient could not name to sound stimulation at all, suggesting a failure of auditory processing; one patient was anomic for smell, but could match smell to picture; all other subjects were closely clustered for all modalities (Goodglass, 1980a,b).

These data argue for the existence of a supramodal "concept" as a first access step in naming. However, naming is slower for all subjects for smell and sound stimulation than for picture and touch. This suggests that the richer a sensory input is, the more effective it is in arousing concepts. (Smell and sound are impoverished in dimensions of experience; vision and touch give texture, size, shape, and other information.)

Bisiach (1966) showed that patients named better if given a full-color picture than if given an outline, and better if given a good outline than a degraded outline—yet they were able to show they knew what the objects were even when they were unable to name. North (1971) also argues that concept arousal is dependent on the redundancy of the input. She created impoverished visual stimuli by blurring the focus on slides until only 90 percent of pilot subjects could identify the objects pictured, and she created a tactile "blur" by wrapping objects in thin layers of foam rubber until the same 90 percent criterion was met. She then presented these "blurred" stimuli to anomic patients and replicated Bisiach's findings; she also showed that anomics retrieved names better when shown the blurred slides and given the wrapped object together than when they were presented with either degraded stimulus alone.

Let us turn now to attempts to explore the nature of the central concept. Goodglass and Baker (1976) attempted to measure the status of various patients' semantic representation by studying their ability to recognize whether certain words (presented auditorily) were associates of a target word (presented as a picture). For example, with the target "orange" the patients heard a variety of nonassociated words mixed in with such associates as "apple," "fruit," "juicy," "eat," "breakfast," and "orange" itself. It was shown that aphasics with comprehension disorders of different severity

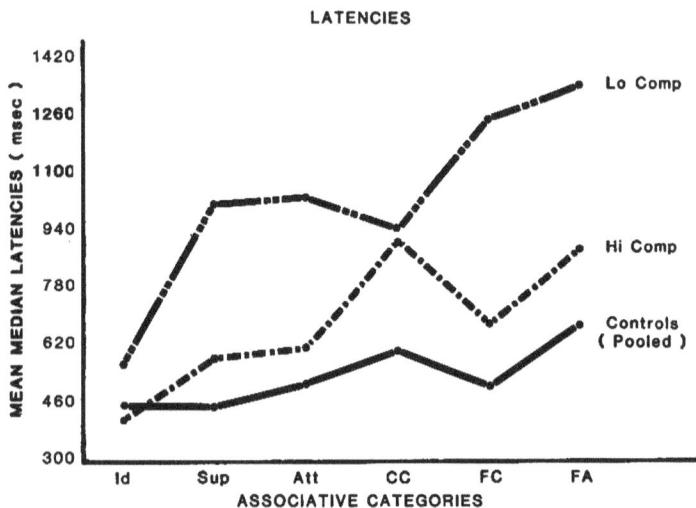

23A

Figure 23.
(*A*) Mean response latencies to associative categories. (*B*) Mean percentage error rate (failure to respond) to associative categories. (Goodglass and Baker, 1976)

gave different patterns of response, both in latency for responding to recognized associates and in failures to recognize the association at all (figure 23).

High-comprehension aphasics looked much like normals; low-comprehension aphasics were similar to these other subjects in two categories, namely, identity (orange-orange) and contrast coordinate (orange-apple). The notion that the integrity of the field of associates of a concept may facilitate naming is supported by the fact that failure to name an object was heavily correlated with failure to recognize many of the words associated with it.

Let us proceed to the next stage in naming. If there has been some degree of arousal of the concept, will there be retrieval of phonological information? If Broca's aphasics

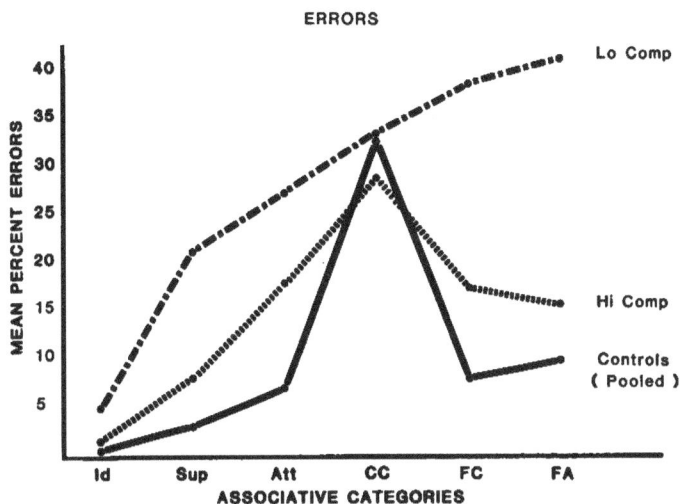

ERRORS

23B

fail primarily at this downstream stage of production—which is suggested by the fact that they respond well to cuing with the first few sounds of the word—they should have good tacit knowledge of the word's phonology. The same should be true of conduction aphasics, whose errors in naming show a general sense of the shape of a word and who reject their own failed attempts.

These hypotheses have been tested with tip-of-the-tongue studies, studies of response to different types of cuing (Pease and Goodglass, 1978), and studies of the recognition of homonyms and rhymes (Kohn, Schonle, and Hawkins, 1982).

In the tip-of-the-tongue (TOT) study (Goodglass et al., 1976), clear cases of anomic, Wernicke's, Broca's, and conduction aphasics were used. When they failed to name pictures presented to them, they were asked to show the number of syllables in the name (having been trained how to do this

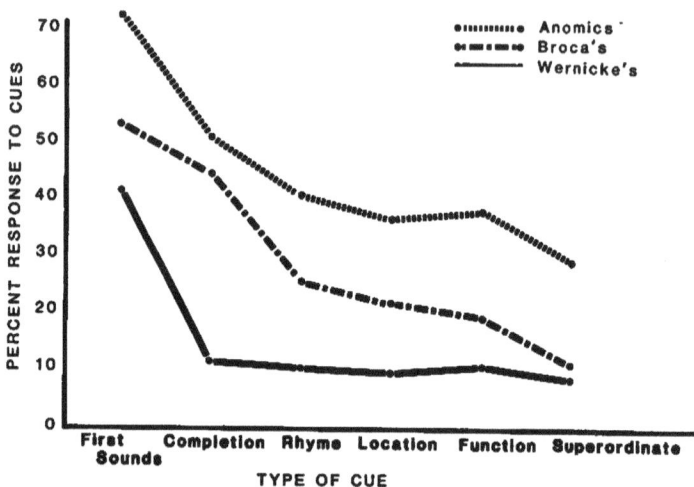

Figure 24.
Percentage of correct responses to each cue category for subjects in three diagnostic categories. (Pease and Goodglass, 1978)

before the experiment) and to indicate the first letter of the name. This study gave some—but only partial—support to the notion of naming stages. Conduction aphasics showed considerable knowledge of the sound of words they could not name, while Wernicke's aphasics did not, as hypothesized; but Broca's aphasics also did poorly, which was unexpected.

In a further study, Pease and Goodglass (1978) observed the effectiveness of different types of cues (initial sound, rhyme, location, function, superordinate) for different types of aphasics and showed that the only cue that helped Wernicke's aphasics was the initial sound of the word (figure 24). In this experiment aphasia type and severity were confounded; but in a later study Goodglass and Stuss (1979) showed that Broca's aphasics benefited more than anomics and Wernicke's aphasics from priming with the first sound, even allowing for severity.

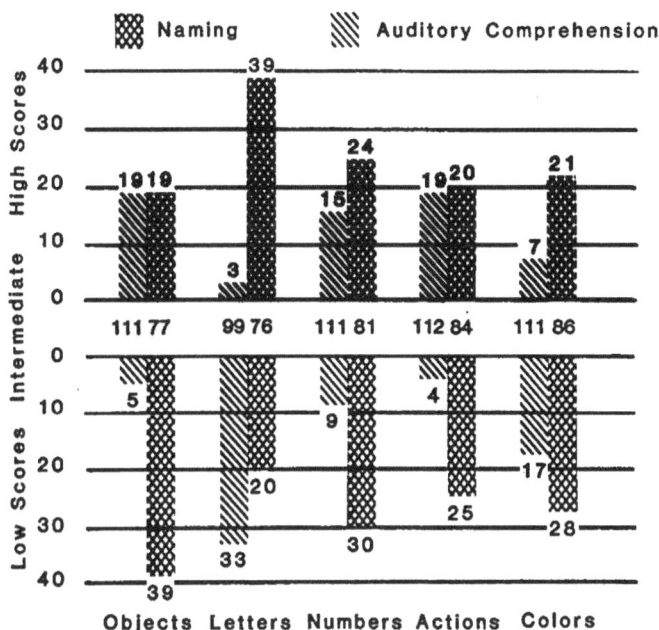

Figure 25.
Distribution of naming and auditory comprehension scores for
five classes of stimuli; responses of 135 aphasics of all types.
High scores indicate preserved ability; low scores, impairment.
(Goodglass, 1980a)

Preliminary work on a homonym- or rhyme-selection test using pictures has given some puzzling results; one severe Wernicke's aphasic with very paraphasic speech performed well on this task. More expectedly, perfect performance on selection of pictures of objects with homonymous names and of pictures of objects with rhyming names was produced by a Broca's aphasic with good comprehension and virtually no speech output.

Finally, we should discuss the dissociation of the ability to name from the ability to recognize the names of different categories such as colors, letters, actions, and object names (figure 25). We note some selective preservations and selective impairments of one or another of the dissociated abilities—for example, in naming, the naming of objects is commonly the worst area of performance and the naming of letters is commonly spared, while in comprehension, the recognition of names of letters is commonly the worst. Various factors, such as the size of the set, the mode of learning, and the characteristics of the sound patterns of the words, have been suggested to account for this pattern of dissociations, but none is fully satisfactory to date. One patient was selectively very poor in the comprehension of both letter names and body-part names, yet was able to name them all. This is difficult to deal with in terms of a model in which production and comprehension of words are each governed by the central representation of the lexical item.

Comments

The question was raised as to how far it might be useful, in some of the cases described by Benson and Goodglass, to draw on a distinction between the abstract phonological representation of a word and its articulatory, or phonetic, execution. Were there perhaps occasions when an aphasic speaker, stymied for a word, had its phonological representation, but not its phonetic?—rather like the so-called deep dyslexic who reads *cat* as *dog*, demonstrating that he has accessed the correct semantic field (perhaps by means of the word's alphabetical phonological representation), but cannot implement the rules that would carry him to the phonetic surface. (Whether, indeed, the "deep dyslexic" has a phonological representation rather than a gross visual association, like someone who can "read" nothing except the names written on public buildings, such as *bank* and *post office*, is, of course, an open question.)

In any event, it would seem that cases certainly do occur, notably perhaps among Broca's aphasics, in which a phonological-to-phonetic break has occurred. A clear example is provided by individuals who can write the name of an object, but cannot say it.

However, it is evident that naming disorders typically run deeper than this. The burden of these two reports is, in fact, one of caution. The hierarchy (and diversity) of naming disorders, outlined by Benson, and the frequently ambiguous outcome of meticulous tests of a commonsense model of the naming process, described by Goodglass, demonstrate that we do not yet even have a viable and coherent description of the lexicon or the processes of word retrieval. Perhaps this is not surprising, since it is precisely at the level of the lexicon that language makes contact with nonlinguistic cognition. In fact, although there is an encouraging degree of overlap between lesion sites that produce naming deficits and stimulation sites found by Ojemann to block naming (see his chapter in part II), there is evidently substantial overlap with neuroanatomical areas that subserve other functions; the angular gyrus, for example (where, incidentally, Ojemann was *not* able to produce an effect), is evidently essential to both linguistic and nonlinguistic modes. Yet, even at the level of behavior *within* the linguistic system, Goodglass cannot find unequivocal support for what would appear to be a minimal requirement, namely, a single representation for both input and output of a single lexical item.

In short, the facts of naming disorders certainly support the notion of functional specialization within the brain, but do not encourage a view of naming as unitary, holistic, or autonomous.

Issues Regarding Vocabulary Skills in Aphasia

E. B. Zurif

This discussion of vocabulary problems in aphasia bears upon two aspects: one, whether language can be viewed as an isolable and neurologically independent cognitive system; and two, the locus of the disruption to vocabulary skills in the various aphasias.

I. There are those who have argued that it is misleading to characterize the effects of left-hemispheric damage in linguistic and psycholinguistic terms and have claimed instead that language is dependent on the left hemisphere just to the extent that it has certain properties and demands certain processing capacities in common with other activities for which this hemisphere is specialized. One version of this argument—popularly held by "holistic" neurologists (Head, 1926; Goldstein, 1948; Bay, 1964)—is that the left hemisphere is a "symbolic" hemisphere and that damage to it also affects other symbolic activities. In this view, aphasia and purposive movement disorders are considered to be two reflections of an underlying "asymbolia."

There is some justification for this view. Aphasia does frequently cooccur with disruptions in the ability to perform object-associated, or object-referable, gestures in the absence of the object—disruptions, for example, in the ability to pantomime what one does with, how one uses, a hammer. And, intuitively, there is some symbolic similarity between pantomimic capacity of this sort and the capacity to refer verbally to objects. That is, it seems reasonable to suppose that both capabilities contact a level of representation at which referential meaning is embedded in the complex matrix of properties and relations that structure our knowledge about objects.

But having registered this support for asymbolia, I hasten to delimit it by emphasizing that so far as language is concerned, my remarks have encompassed only one language activity: naming—that is, the ability to identify and to produce distinctive responses to refer to objects and events. And in most views, such activity is hardly the hallmark of language; rather, it is to be found in many uninstructed, naturally acquired symbol systems, including symbolic attire, facial expressions, and folkloric painting idioms (see the chapter by M. Liberman).

Indeed, when the domain of inquiry is widened to include not just vocabulary but, more generally, the processing of *sentence* form and meaning (that is, to include structures and procedures more likely to be dissimilar to those involved in other cognitive activities), then the relation between pantomimic activity and aphasia becomes less certain. Specifically, although the two often cooccur, the presence of the movement disorder does not reliably predict either the severity of the aphasia or its clinical form (Goodglass and Kaplan, 1963). In short, the form of the *grammatical* disruption seems exempt from the correlation.

Even then, under the most rudimentary of functional analyses—even if the distinction between word meaning and sentence form (phonology and syntax) is drawn in the broadest of terms—it still seems reasonable to suggest the existence of neural mechanisms uniquely implicated in the exercise of language.

II. The concern here is with determining the locus of the disruption that underlies naming and word-comprehension disorders in aphasia. Roughly, the issue is to determine whether the organization of semantic storage is somehow deficient (see the chapter by Caplan in this part)—or whether the problem is with the mechanisms that retrieve or address this stored information.

Consider word comprehension: One effort—particularly concerned to account for lexical comprehension in Wernicke's aphasia, where the problem is most acute—has sought to implicate initial (access) disruptions within what seems to be a serial processing framework (Luria, 1970). The argument here runs that the semantic representation for a word would be found intact if only the acoustic input could be properly coded for the purpose of addressing the semantic lexicon. Yet, notwithstanding that Wernicke's area is adjacent to auditory cortex and that lesions to this area might thereby disrupt acoustic analysis, recent work has indicated that even if there are disruptions at the initial processing stages, they cannot straightforwardly account for the Wernicke's aphasic's lexical comprehension problem (see, for example, Baker, Blumstein, and Goodglass, 1981). Rather, there seems to be a complicated interaction involving "top-down" effects, so that as semantic discriminations increase in difficulty, phoneme discrimination is adversely affected.

In like fashion, production problems—that is, word-finding difficulties—also resist explanations that turn solely on "access" deficits, that is, on deficits in retrieving lexical forms from a preserved memory for semantic structures. Those who stress access problems (for example, Weigl-Crump and Koenigsknecht, 1973) point to the clinical facts of variability in naming performance (Goodglass and Geschwind, 1976), the success of phonetic cuing, and the occasional instances of vocabulary recovery, the (usually implicit) assumption being that an immutable limitation or dislocation of stored semantic information would disallow such effects. This implicit assumption may be far from correct, however. Dislocation to semantic structure or even partial erasure of semantic information could also be implicated in an account of these facts; quite simply, success in retrieving a phonetic response via the semantic representation could as easily depend on the extent of the damage to the storage system as on the status of the retrieval mechanisms.

This argument can be made more explicit by considering studies relating naming to perceptual processing. Briefly, it has been observed that aphasic patients, especially Wernicke's aphasic patients, have a less than normal ability to integrate the sensory properties of objects to be named (Bisiach, 1966; North, 1971). The lesson to be taken from this finding seemed, at first, to be rather straightforward; it seemed reasonable to suppose that the underlying semantic representation of a word remains intact under conditions of brain damage, but that it is insufficiently activated via sensory information from the object to be named and so cannot be used to access the word. This view now appears less tenable, however. Again, a top-down effect cannot be ruled out; problems in integrating the sensory information inherent in an object to be named cannot be so easily divorced from a disruption to the manner in which perceptual and functional information is structured at the semantic level.

Of relevance here is a model of naming currently being elaborated by Caramazza and his colleagues, Berndt and Brownell (Caramazza et al., 1982). The initial stages of this model include a *semantically* constrained parsing of the perceptual input; faced with the object, "cup," for example, the output of the parser might be expected to isolate the semantically interpretable feature "handle." This model allows the prediction that since perceptual parsing for the purpose of categorization is guided by semantic considerations, disruption at the lexical semantic level will manifest itself, not as a sensory deficit, but rather as an impairment in the *perceptual isolation* of semantically interpretable components. And on such evidence as is available, this seems to be the case: Patients who had problems naming objects were also impaired in their judgments of perceptual similarity of these objects, *even apart from naming*. Since all the patients tested were screened on their ability to group perceptually shapes of different sizes and colors—that is, since there were no indications of strictly perceptual deficits—it seems reasonable to assume that the deficit is at the level of the semantic representation of the perceptual information, the level that defines the categories tested.

Finally, and to implicate yet again the lexical-semantic level in the aphasic vocabulary disorder, a number of recent investigations point to a connection between, on the one hand, the ability of aphasic patients to find and to understand words and, on the other hand, their ability to trace conceptual relations among words (see, for example, Goodglass and Baker, 1976; Zurif et al., 1974).

Acknowledgment

Some of the work reported here was supported by NIH grants 11408, 15972, and 06209.

PART IV

Syntax as an Autonomous Component of Language

Z. W. Pylyshyn

Resolving the issue of whether syntax is an autonomous component of language hinges on what is meant by "syntax." It is a mistake to think that the intuitive notion of syntax is appropriate. To be a natural domain of study the concept of "syntactic rule" must be characterized technically. This characterization must describe the properties of language as a *coding system*. In other words, the theory of syntax appraises the *structure* of a sentence as distinct from the *content* of that sentence. Thus, knowledge of syntax is only one part of linguistic knowledge and is clearly insufficient to motivate every inference that may be drawn from a sentence. But it should suffice to discriminate sentence meanings and to account in part for our ability to generate novel acceptable sentences. Syntax provides the resources for forming semantic distinctions using the lexicon and grammatical devices.

It is assumed that syntactic coding has a structure and that this structure can be described. The autonomy issue does not depend simply on this assertion, of course, but on a more fundamental empirical question: Is there a part of the cognitive system that exclusively computes syntactic forms and performs its computations independent of other knowledge and beliefs about the world?

Were we to follow the grammar school notion of syntax, we would have to conclude that syntax was not autonomous because the acceptability of sentences for a prescriptive grammar *does* depend on knowledge. For example, which of the following two sentences is "grammatically" correct?

I don't know how to choose $\begin{Bmatrix} \text{among} \\ \text{between} \end{Bmatrix}$ P.

This question can only be resolved if we know about P (which might even be an arbitrary predicate in number theory). But this is not the province of syntax; the choice between "between" and "among" only seems to be syntactic because that is what we were taught. It is not a syntactic choice in the technical sense because it depends on knowledge of the world.

A more subtle misunderstanding of the boundaries of syntax was contributed by proponents of generative semantics. They asserted that syntax and meaning could not be separated and that acceptability judgments are always based on syntax and on meaning. For example, consider

1. Mary has a baby and the baby is asleep.

2. Mary's baby is asleep and Mary has a baby.

Native speakers generally accept sentence 1 but reject sentence 2. But it would be futile to capture this distinction in terms of grammatical rules. The acceptability of sentence 2 is a pragmatic issue, germane to communicative practices, irrelevant to syntax; sentence 2 simply violates a norm of conversation (go from the general to the specific).

For syntax to be a useful concept, we must draw the boundary around syntax, so that the structure of the code is independent of commonsense knowledge of the world and conversational rules. We shall then be in a position to test the viability of the concept empirically. Otherwise the strategy of "divide and conquer" will fail.

So what linguists do is prime the pump with clear cases and hope to decompose the system into modules. But we should be clear that the precise characterizations of the syntactic module have changed and will continue to change. Chomsky (1980), for example, has claimed that the syntactic module produces "logical forms" that enter into a system of inference, as in predicate calculus. There is reason to doubt that this can be precisely the case, however, because some properties of anaphoric reference and quantification scope depend on knowledge of the world. Hence the complete "logical form," with bound variables (in the sense used in predicate calculus) is unlikely to be the output of the syntax module in all cases. What, precisely, the output is remains an active research problem.

Is there psychological evidence for the *reflexive* nature of syntactic processing? Twenty years ago the claim was that the cognitive system guided the parsing of a sentence because syntactic analysis is indeterminate. (That is, there are many analyses compatible with a given set of syntactic rules.) If this were true, there would be no independent syntactic processing component. However, within the last fifteen years (Fodor, Bever, and Garrett, 1974; Forster, 1979; Swinney, 1982; Cairns, in press) evidence has accumulated to indicate that parsing *is* an automatic (or what some people call reflexive) phenomenon.

This automaticity seems to extend to lexical activities as well. As an example of the latter, consider an experimental task in which a subject must name the color of the ink a word is printed in. If the word itself is a color name, performance is degraded when ink color and word mismatch (Stroop, 1935), though the subject is instructed to ignore the word and concentrate on the ink. In an analogous grammatical circumstance, experiments have studied performance when subjects are instructed to ignore the grammatical structure and meaning of sentences. These studies show, for example, that the ease of detecting a particular phoneme in fluent speech varies as a function of grammatical structure (Foss, 1969), even when subjects deliberately ignore sentence structure and meaning.

Arguments against autonomy usually concentrate on the nondeterministic properties of grammatical rules (Schank, 1972). For any sentence there may be multiple structural interpretations, each compatible with the grammar, and we do not seem to be aware of this multiplicity during sentence perception. This seems to show that there has been cognitive intervention. However, careful experiments reveal that we do *not* make decisions about meaning until after the syntactic analysis has been performed without benefit of cognitive intervention (Forster, 1979). Phoneme monitoring is hampered when a sentence is syntactically ambiguous (Foss, 1970).

Lexical priming also operates in this modular manner (Swinney, 1979). In general, the latency for a lexical decision (did the experimenter just show me a word or a nonword?) may be shortened if the target word is preceded by a related, priming word. The prime presumably facilitates access to the target. Suppose a prime word has two meanings, for example, "bug" (which can mean insect or spying device). Do all associates become primed, or only associates of the meaning that was actually understood? Swinney forced subjects to adopt a particular meaning of a potentially ambiguous word by presenting the prime in a strongly biasing sentence context.

They found several spiders, roaches and other *bugs* in the room.

They uncovered several microphones transmitters and other *bugs* in the room.

Perhaps unexpectedly, each meaning of "bug" primed associates of both the correct homograph and the other, unnoticed homograph. Lexical decision latencies to both ANT and SPY were shortened regardless of which meaning of the prime was heard in the disambiguated context.

To conclude, much of linguistic analysis appears to be an "ignorant" process, though its isolation from knowledge of the world does not render computer implementation of syntactic processes particularly tractable. Machines such as computers have very different architecture from machines such as brains. A computing machine with a different type of architecture than the computers we presently possess might permit an easier simulation than is now possible.

Comments

In subsequent discussion. Pylyshyn remarked that the attempt to decompose language into a set of cognitively impenetrable functions was justified on both methodological and substantive grounds. Methodologically, the strategy is one of divide and conquer, on the assumption that if we can find separable domains, we shall have a better chance of understanding the whole system. Substantively, the hypothesis of cognitively impenetrable functions, or modules, explicitly recognizes that the task of cognitive psychology is to explain cognition in terms of more primitive noncognitive mechanisms, splitting the system into a set of automatic mechanisms from which the capacities of the whole system may ultimately be seen to emerge. These impenetrable mechanisms are the functional architecture of the system, the biological resources from which the system is constructed. The distance between cognition and neurophysiology is greatest when we attempt to deal with the general, commonsense reasoning part of the language system (where all the plasticity lies), least when we deal with its modular components. Our best chance of capturing the interface between biology and cognition may lie in the neurophysiological modeling of these modular components.

Language Structure and Language Breakdown in American Sign Language

U. Bellugi

I. Structure of Sign Language

A. Sublexical Structure

Current research has shown that signed languages, like spoken languages, display a dual pattern of both phonology (or sign-formational structure) and syntax. In spoken language, the basic meaningful units are constructed from a small set of arbitrary and meaningless elements arranged in linear contrasts to form morphemes and words. The contrasting elements and the rules for combining them differ from language to language, but the division into a small set of meaningless elements that combine in rule-governed ways to form a vast and open meaningful vocabulary is universal across languages.

Like the words of spoken languages, signs of American Sign Language (ASL) are fractionated into sublexical elements. The component parameters of signs are different from those of words; signs are constituted by configurations of the hand or hands, places of articulation, and movements (Stokoe, Casterline, and Croneberg, 1976). The number of possible configurations the hand can physically assume, the number of possible places of articulation, the number of possible kinds of movement is very large indeed. Yet ASL uses only a limited set of formational components—a set similar in size to the limited set of phonemes posited for spoken languages. Further, as with spoken languages, there are systematic restrictions on the ways these components can combine (Klima and Bellugi, 1979).

Observational, historical, and experimental evidence support this structural view of signs. The sublexical parameters constrain new signs as they enter ASL as borrowings and account for their diminishing iconicity over time (Bellugi and Newkirk, 1980; Frishberg, 1975). The processing and rehearsal of signs in short-term memory is clearly in terms of the formational components (Bellugi, Klima, and Siple, 1975; Poizner, Bellugi, and Tweney, 1981). Slips of the hand (analogous to slips of the tongue) involve substitutions of component elements of signs, and the resulting misordering of elements involves systematically predicted combinations of elements (Newkirk et al., 1980). Signers are aware of the internal structure of signs; they substitute and make use of the component elements in plays on signs and in creating poetic sign form (using, for example, one handshape throughout a line of poetry as a kind of alliteration). Such deliberate manipulation of elements of the linguistic system clearly reflects the intuitive awareness of linguistic form (Klima and Bellugi, 1976).

The formational components and their combinatorial possibilities differ from one sign language to another. Comparison of two different sign languages with independent histories, Chinese Sign Language and American Sign Language, shows once again a parallelism with spoken languages; the two different sign languages have different inventories of components, and even when the component elements are the same, there are differing restrictions on their combination into morphemes (Klima and Bellugi, 1979). Studies of the formational components of other sign languages (Ahlgren and Bergman, 1980; Frokjaer-Jensen, 1980) confirm these findings.

All these results indicate that the formational parameters of signs have psychological as well as linguistic significance.

B. Three-dimensional Morphology

At all levels, there are grammmatical devices in ASL that are analogous in function to those of spoken language (Klima and Bellugi, 1979; Lane and Grosjean, 1980; Liddell, 1980; Siple, 1978; Wilbur, 1979; Baker and Cokely, 1980; Bellugi and Klima, 1980; Bellugi and Studdert-Kennedy, 1980; Bellugi, 1980a; Newport and Supalla, 1980; Newport, in press). American Sign Language is clearly a fully expressive language, with grammatical structuring like that of spoken languages. But some of the formal devices that ASL has developed make use of possibilities either not available or not so used in the vocal-auditory modality of spoken languages.

Like spoken languages, ASL has developed grammatical markers that function as inflectional and derivational morphemes, resulting in regular changes in form across syntactic classes of lexical items that produce systematic changes in meaning. The elaborate system of formal inflectional devices, their widespread use to vary the form of signs, and the variety of fine distinctions they systematically convey suggest that ASL, like, say, Russian and Navajo, is one of the inflective languages of the world.

Verb signs, for instance, undergo obligatory inflections for indexic reference that identify the arguments of the verb; for reciprocity (for example, 'to each other'); for several distinctions of grammatical number (for example, 'to both,' 'to more than two'); for distinctions of distributional aspect (for example, 'to each,' 'to any,' 'to certain ones at different times'); for distinctions of temporal aspect (for example, 'for a long time,' 'over and over again,' 'uninterruptedly,' 'regularly'); for distinctions of temporal focus (for example, 'starting to,' 'increasingly,' 'resulting in'); for distinctions of manner (for example, 'with ease,' 'approximately'). Figure 26 shows an array of such inflectional operations on the single sign root ASK.[1] Some are inflections for temporal aspect and focus and for distributional aspect, marking modulations of meaning such as recurrence of events over time, distribution of action across events. There is also a large number of derivational processes, such as those that form deverbal nouns; nominalizations of verbs; derivation of predicates from nouns; and derivations for extended or figurative meaning. Each morphological process embeds a sign stem in a distinctive superimposed dynamic spatial contour of movement, leaving other structural parameters (handshape, target locus) intact.

In ASL inflectional processes can apply in combinations to root signs, creating different hierarchies of form and meaning. In these combinations the output of one inflectional process serves as the input for another, and there are alternative orderings with different hierarchies of semantic structure as well. Such hierarchical organization and recursive application of rules to create complex expressions are also characteristic of spoken-language structure. The proliferation of cooccurring components in spatial patterning brought into play at the morphological level and in the language in general is consistent with our view of the tendency of the language toward conflation: toward packaging a great deal of information systematically in cooccurring layers of structure (Bellugi and Klima, 1980).

In some respects the morphology of American Sign Language resembles that of Semitic languages. It may be instructive to examine some of their similarities and differences. In a Semitic language such as Hebrew, there are large sets of words related in form and meaning. These can be characterized as combinations of two types of elements: consonantal roots and morphological patterns, the latter consisting of discontinuous vowel sequences and sometimes including one or more prefixes and/or suffixes. It has been argued that these are appropriately analyzed as multitiered structures (McCarthy, 1979). The root is considered as one tier consisting of consonants, and inflectional and derivational morphemes as another tier. For example, the root k-t-v is considered to be the basis for such words as *katav*, 'write';

UNINFLECTED FORM:

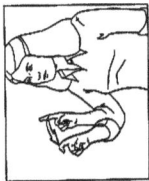

ASK (Uninflected)

REFERENTIAL INDEXING:

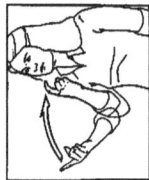

ASK [Indexic: 1st Pers.]
'ask me'

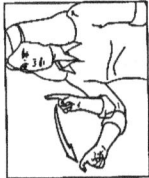

ASK [Indexic: 2nd Pers.]
'ask you'

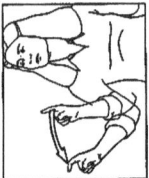

ASK [Indexic: 3rd Pers.]
'ask him'

GRAMMATICAL NUMBER:

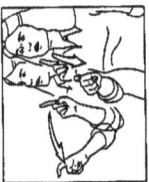

ASK [Dual]
'ask both'

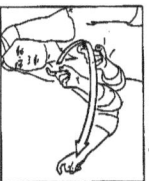

ASK [Multiple]
'ask them'

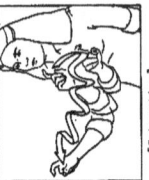

ASK [Exhaustive]
'ask each of them'

RECIPROCAL:

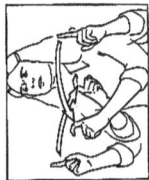

ASK [Reciprocal]
'ask each other'

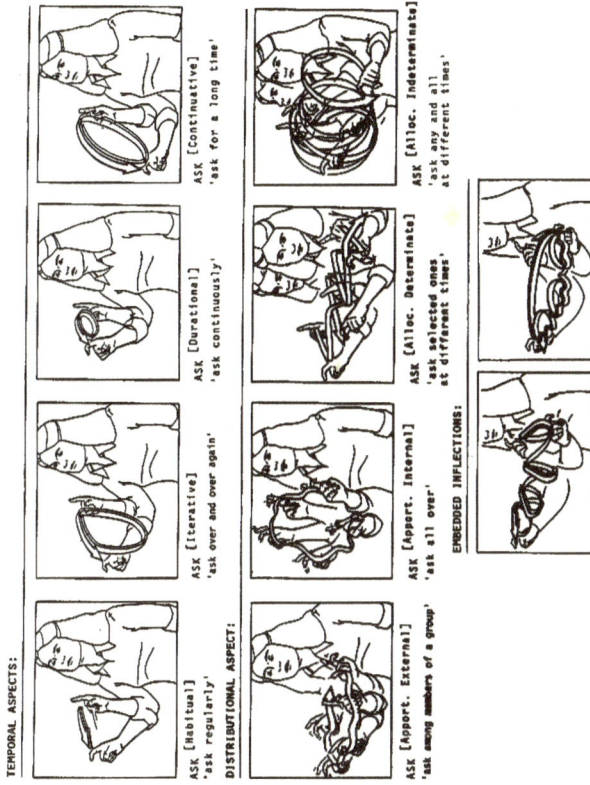

Figure 26.
Inflectional operations on a single root. (Bellugi)

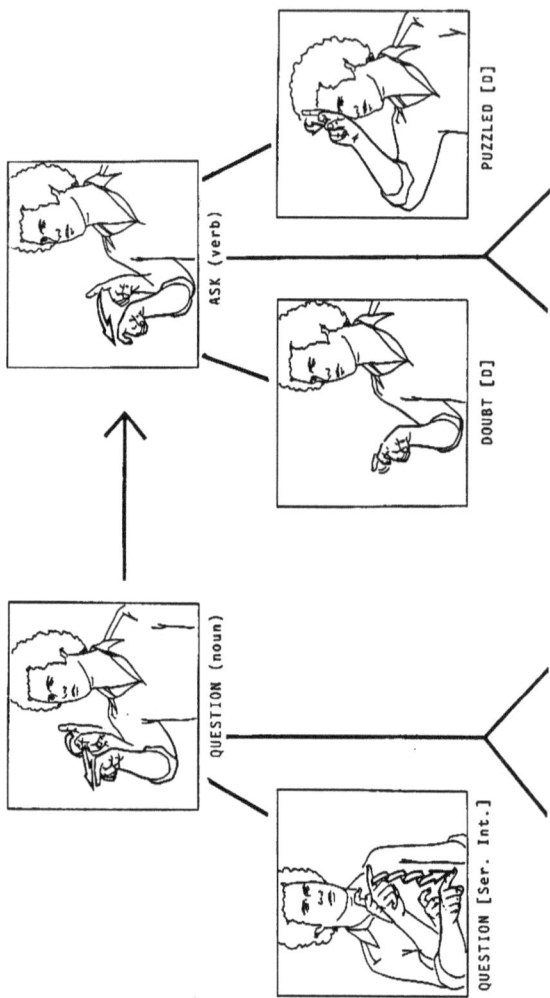

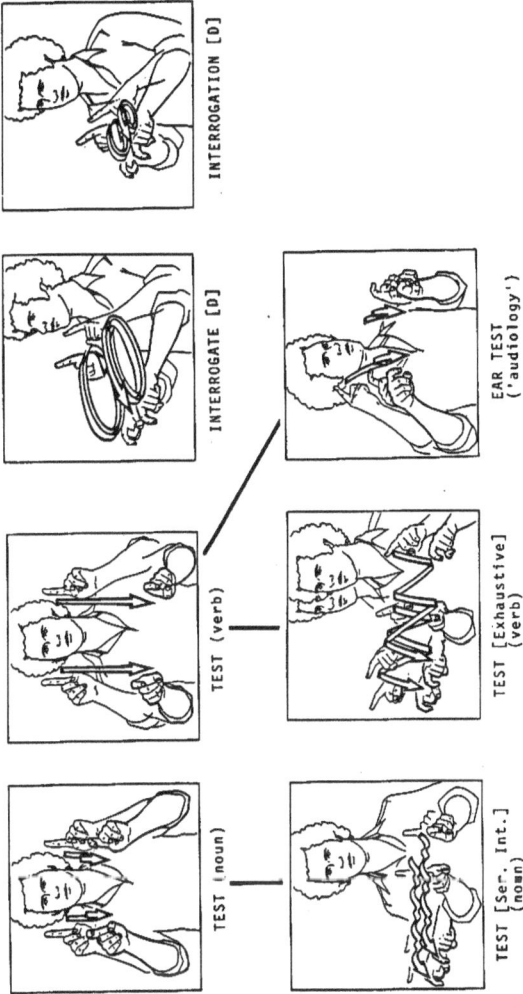

Figure 27.
ASK/QUESTION and some related forms. (Bellugi, 1982)

ktiv, 'spelling'; *ktav*, 'script'; *katuv*,'written'; *katava*, 'news-report'; *hitkatev*, 'correspond'; and so forth (Berman, 1978). The surface form is realized as the intercalation of vowels and additional consonants with the root form. In languages like the Semitic languages, there is no structural justification for considering the surface form as a root preceded or followed by a prefix or suffix. According to some current considerations of universal grammar, languages like English are special cases in which the inflectional/derivational tiers happen to be spelled out as contiguous units, typically as prefixes or suffixes (Halle and Vergnaud, 1980).

In a sign language like ASL, there are also large sets of forms that are related in form and meaning. We have argued that the appropriate analysis of these morphological structures in ASL is also in terms of multiple tiers. There is an underlying root, and overlaid concurrently with it are derivational and inflectional tiers. Looking over the set of forms presented in figures 26 and 27, for example, notice that they all share certain properties of hand configuration and local movement as the basis for a wide variety of surface forms, for example, those meaning 'ask me,' 'ask you,' 'ask each other,' 'ask each of them,' 'ask regularly,' 'ask all over,' 'ask easily,' 'doubt,' 'puzzled,' 'test,' 'question,' 'interrogate,' 'interrogation,' 'inquire,' 'inquisition.' According to one view, the root of this family of forms is a /G/ handshape and a closing (local) movement of the index finger. Inflectional and derivational processes represent the interaction of this root with other features of movement in space (manners of movement, direction of movement, dynamics, and the like). For example, the form ASK is a /G/ handshape closing while moving forward; the related verb TEST is a /G/ handshape closing while moving downward with hold manner; the related noun TEST is a /G/ handshape closing while moving downward with restrained manner, duplicated. Note that unlike the examples from Hebrew, the surface forms of ASL inflectional and derivational patterns may retain their tiered structure in the final output, and yet the regularities that relate root and morphologically complex forms—the formal rules—are similar in the two types of languages.

Syntactic Spatial Mechanisms

Languages have different ways of marking grammatical relations among their lexical items. In English, basic grammatical relations among verbs and their arguments are signaled largely by the order of items; in other languages these relations are signaled by case marking or verb agreement morphology. All of these rely on linear ordering of words or segments. By contrast, in a visual-spatial language like American Sign Language, relations among signs are stipulated primarily by manipulation of sign forms in space. A horizontal plane in front of the signer's torso plays an important role in the structure of the language, not simply as an articulatory space for hand and arm movements comparable to the mouth cavity for the tongue, but also as a carrier of linguistic meaning. (For discussion of spatial syntactic mechanisms, see Padden, 1979, 1981, 1982.) This emphasizes an essential difference between signed and spoken languages; the spatial domain figures prominently in many aspects of ASL structure.

Nominals introduced into the discourse are associated with specific points in a plane of signing space. Pointing to a specific locus later in the discourse clearly refers back to a specific nominal, even after many intervening signs. Such spatial indexing allows explicit coreference and reduces the possibility of ambiguity. The English sentence, "He said he hit him and then he fell down" does not specify which, if any, of the pronoun instances are coreferential. In ASL such distinctions are obligatory and are made by indexing different points in space.

The system of verb agreement in ASL, like the pronominal system, is essentially spatialized; verb signs move between abstract loci in signing space. Verbs like ASK, INFORM,

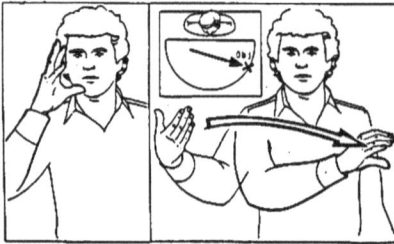

MOTHER   ₃ᵢFORCE₃ⱼ

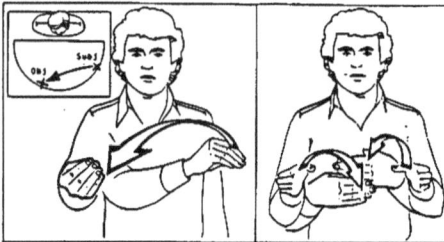

₃ⱼGIVE₃ₖ   BOX

28A

Figure 28.
Spatial syntactic mechanisms of American Sign Language.
(*A*) 'Mother forced him to give someone the box.' (*B*) Diagram
of verb complement embedding. (*C*) Diagrams of multiple and
embedded spaces. (Padden, 1982)

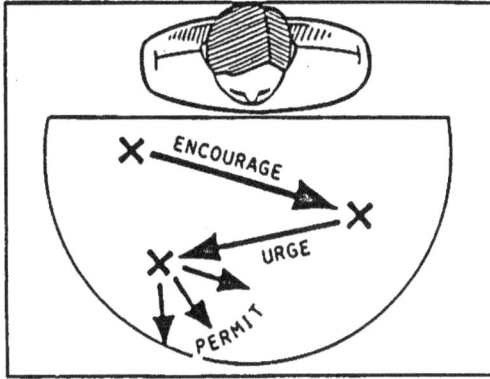

28B

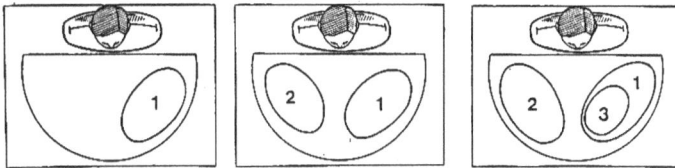

28C

GIVE are obligatorily marked for person (and number) via spatial indices. The indices dictate the verb's path (the initial and final points) from one indexic locus to the other and specify the subject and object of the verb. Thus the same signs, in the same order, but with a change in direction of movement of the verb, indicate different grammatical relations. Furthermore, meaning can be preserved under a different temporal order of signs, since relations are specified spatially. The system of spatial indexing permits relative freedom of word order (in simple sentences, anyway) and yet provides clear specification of grammatical relations by spatial means.

Coreferential nominals must be indexed to the same locus point, as is evident in embedded structures. In complement structures with matrix verbs like FORCE, URGE, PERSUADE, the direct object of the matrix clause must be identical with the subject of the embedded clause. Thus in the sentence illustrated in figure 28A, the spatial points for matrix direct object and embedded subject must be identical. The unique kind of special organization involved in ASL sentences can be seen in sentences with multiclausal embedding. For a sentence like the following, the locus points specify sentential relations. (see figure 28B):

$_1$ENCOURAGE$_{3i}$ $_{3i}$URGE$_{3j}$ $_{3j}$PERMIT$_{3k}$ $^{[Exhaustive]}$ TAKE-UP CLASS

'I encouraged her to urge him to permit each of them to take the class.'

Note that in these complex sentences the set of possible spatial points is severely constrained.

The space used by the signer is partitioned in very special ways. The specific horizontal plane in front of the signer's torso is the locus for indices of definite reference, that is, when the speaker has a referent in mind that he introduces into the discourse. Different spaces can be used for contrasting events, for indicating reference to time prior to the utterance, for hypotheticals and counterfactuals. It is possible even to embed smaller subspaces within one subspace, for example, as in embedding a conditional subspace within a past time context. (see figure 28C).

Clearly the use of space in all the different systems briefly mentioned here (pronominal reference, verb agreement, coreferentiality, spatial contexts) is extremely complex and dynamic. In each subsystem there is a mediation between the visual-spatial mode in which the language has developed and the overlaid grammatical constraints in the language. Thus the syntax of American Sign Language relies heavily on manipulation of abstract points in space and of spatial representation. This difference in surface form of syntactic

mechanisms may have important consequences for the
neurobiological substrate of spoken and signed languages.

II. Acquisition of Sign Language by Deaf Children

We have been studying the acquisition of ASL by deaf children of deaf parents. We investigate the processes by which
deaf children master the grammatical properties of the language, intertwining analysis of spontaneous signing at
monthly intervals with controlled testing and experimental
procedures (Bellugi and Klima, 1982a,b; Boyes-Braem, 1981;
Launer, 1982; Loew, 1982; Maxwell, 1980; Meier, 1981,
1982; Newport and Supalla, 1980; Newport and Ashbrook,
1977; Supalla, 1982. See also Hoffmeister, 1975, 1978; Hoffmeister and Wilbur, 1980; Kantor, 1982; McIntire, 1977).

In general, the acquisition process in deaf children of deaf
parents proceeds in a way that is strikingly similar to the
acquisition of spoken language in hearing children. However,
some details are more like the acquisition of Hebrew (which
is a similarly inflective language) than like English (Berman,
1982). In other respects, the fact that it is a visual language
makes certain aspects of ASL acquisition appear different
from spoken language. Specifically, the visual-spatial nature
of the grammar of the language may affect details of the
acquisition process.

Deaf children around the age of two begin with uninflected
signs, even when imitating their mothers' signs and even
where marking for person, number, and so forth is grammatically required in the adult language. By the age of three,
deaf children have learned basic aspects of verb morphology
in ASL (inflections for person, inflections for temporal aspect
and number; see Meier, 1981, 1982).

As noted, in ASL nominals introduced into the discourse
are assigned unique spatial loci; verbs move between such
spatial loci to specify relations between arguments of the
verbs. Young deaf children by the age of three certainly

communicate about what is not present in the immediate context of the discourse; however, they do so using nominal signs not associated with locus points in signing space and without pronominal indices. Sometimes the children index verbs in space but without specifying the nominals established at these loci, and thus the sentences are referentially unclear. Even when deaf children begin indexing verbs to locus points in space, their first attempts do not maintain a one-to-one referent-to-locus mapping. In telling the story of Rapunzel, for example, a child three-and-a-half years old indexed three verbs in space—TAKE (from father); PUSH (to witch); LOOK (at Rapunzel)—yet all were indexed at the same locus. In effect, all three referents (father, witch, Rapunzel) were "stacked up" at a single locus point (Loew, 1982). By the age of five, however, almost every nominal and pronoun is appropriately indexed in space when required, and almost every verb appropriately shows verb agreement, although there are still occasional discourse problems in establishing and maintaining a one-to-one identity mapping for locus points.

It appears that despite the radical difference in modality of language, deaf and hearing children show a similar course of development, given a natural language input at the critical time. The deaf child, as does his hearing counterpart, analyzes out discrete components of the system presented to him. Furthermore, the evidence suggests that even when the modality and the language offer possibilities that seem intuitively obvious (for example, pointing for deictic pronominal reference), he appears to ignore their putative iconicity. The deaf child treats the language input—even when it includes deictic pointing signs—as part of a formal linguistic system (Bellugi and Klima, 1982a,b).

III. Language and Brain Organization

One of the most distinguishing characteristics of the organization of the human brain is the differential functional

specialization of the left and right hemispheres. In most right-·
handed adults, the left cerebral hemisphere is more important
in aspects of speech and language functioning, and the right
hemisphere is more important in the performance of certain
nonlanguage visual-spatial tasks. Evidence for this specialization of function has accumulated in the last century and
comes from a wide variety of sources (behavioral deficits in
neurological disease, anatomical differences, chemical anesthesia of one or the other hemisphere, "split-brain" patients,
and lateralization studies in normals, including behavioral
studies and monitoring of brain activity). The interpretations
of these findings have differed; proposed alternatives include
(a) the motor control of speech; (b) the processing of complex
acoustic information that contains rapid frequency transitions; (c) the perception of temporal sequences; and (d) linguistic processing involved in the grammatical encoding of
information.

Until very recently, evidence concerning the organization
of the human brain for language has come exclusively from
studies of hearing subjects who use spoken language. It has,
in fact, been argued that there is a privileged hearing-language
connection and that the vocal-auditory language modality
is crucial to the specialization of function of the two cerebral
hemispheres in man. Furthermore, both of the major
language-mediating neural structures identified in the brain,
the so-called Broca's and Wernicke's areas, strongly exhibit
speech connections, the former located near that part of the
left hemisphere that controls movements of the vocal tract,
and the latter contiguous to the primary cortical auditory
center.

Congenitally deaf adults who have learned a primary signed
language, but no language through the auditory modality,
offer a privileged testing ground for hypotheses concerning
the nature of cerebral specialization for language and the
role of experience in its development. Do the structural char-

acteristics of a primary language, arising from its transmission modality, affect neural representation in the brain?

A handful of studies has investigated hemispheric specialization for signs of American Sign Language using behavioral methods such as tachistoscopic presentation of signs to right and left visual fields. Both deaf and hearing subjects tend to show right-hemisphere advantage to signs presented statically across studies, as summarized in Poizner and Battison (1980); in only one study (Neville and Bellugi, 1978) was there a left-hemisphere advantage for static signs. Almost without exception (but see Poizner, Battison, and Lane, 1979) these studies have presented signs as photographs or drawings, that is, as still images for identification. However, processing of static visual images may be quite different from processing of moving signs. As Poizner and Battison (1980) conclude, "Because movement is critical to sign languages and temporal variables now seem critical in determining cerebral asymmetries, the effects of various linguistic movements on cerebral asymmetries . . . needs to be a focal point of future experimental research" (p. 98). This line of research is now being actively pursued in several studies in progress.

There have been only a few scattered case reports of sign aphasia, and even the reports that exist are extremely limited due to the particular sensory and language histories of the patients, extreme underreporting of neurological or linguistic testing, misconceptions about the nature of sign language and lack of knowledge about its linguistic structure. Little can be learned about the effects of brain damage on signing in the studies to date because of these limitations. However, one may note that in the studies available, for the most part, left-hemisphere damage appears to lead to some language impairment in right-handed signers (see for reviews Poizner and Battison, 1980; Kimura, 1982).

We have outlined the issues that are relevant for a study of aphasia in a visual-gestural language in Bellugi, Poizner, and Zurif (1982). Currently we are undertaking the first systematic study of the effects of brain damage on cerebral specialization for language and nonlanguage tasks in groups of deaf patients.

We have begun investigations of the language and visual-spatial skills in deaf patients with unilateral left- and right-hemisphere lesions, all of whom were fluent ASL signers before their lesions. Three patients have lesions confined to the left hemisphere, but with different damage. One patient, "Paul," has a left subcortical lesion with damage deep in the frontal lobe and to the parietal lobe. Another patient, "Karen," has left cortical damage primarily to the parietal lobe. A third patient, "Gail," has left cortical lesions involving both the frontal and temporal lobes (encompassing the traditional Broca's area). To evaluate patients' capacities for sign language, we administered a version of the Boston Diagnostic Aphasia Examination (Goodglass and Kaplan, 1972) adapted for use in American Sign Language, as well as specific tests devised for structural layers of the language (sublexical, semantic, morphological, syntactic). Furthermore, we administered a battery of visual-spatial tasks designed to distinguish left- and right-hemisphere damage. (These studies are reported in Padden, Bellugi, and Poizner (1982) and Poizner et al. (1982).)

The three patients' signing performance clearly shows language impairment, although other specific nonlanguage skills were spared. Two patients (Paul and Karen) are still "fluent" signers, even after left hemisphere damage; the third (Gail) is "nonfluent": her signing is characterized by effortful restricted production of limited open class signs, with none of the grammatical apparatus of the language, although she was a fluent ASL signer before her lesion. Furthermore, her visual-spatial skills (drawing, 3-D block construction, WAIS block designs, Rey-Osterreith complex figure, facial recognition, line orientation, and dot localization) are equivalent to those of normal control subjects—not at all impaired. This is striking evidence that left-hemisphere lesions can lead to sign-

Sign Aphasic

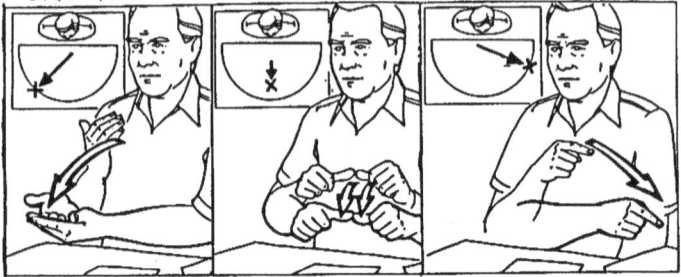

Correct Forms for Context

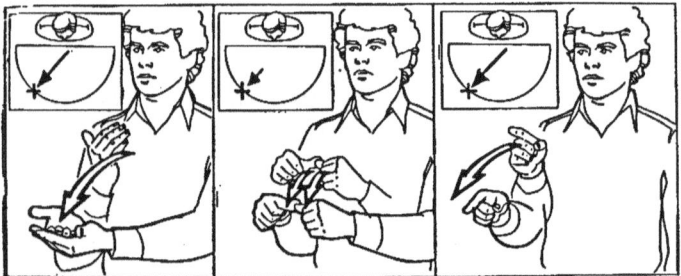

29A

Figure 29.
Language and brain organization: evidence from aphasia. (*A*)
Failure to maintain spatial indices. (*B*) Paragrammaticisms.
(Bellugi)

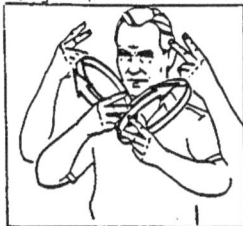 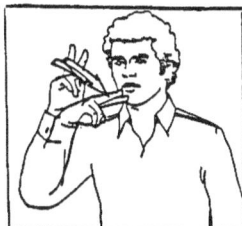

CARELESS [Predispositional]   CARELESS(uninflected)
   'prone to be careless'

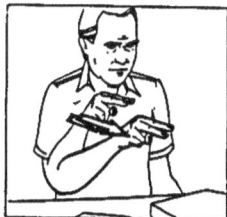 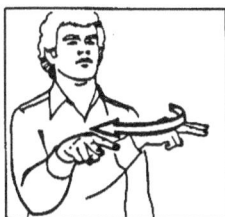

SEE [Habitual]   SEE [Multiple]
'see regularly'   'see them'

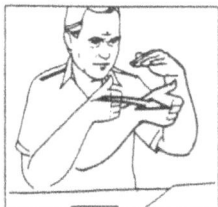 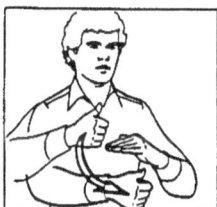

UNDER [Idiomatic Derivative]   UNDER
   'subordinate'

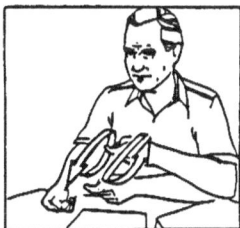 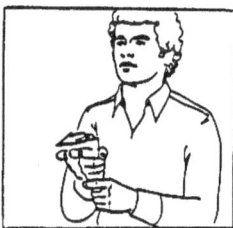

HURT [Derivative]   HURT
   'hazing'

29B

language impairment that is agrammatical but with clear sparing of nonlanguage visual-spatial functions.

The other two patients (Paul and Karen) are fluent signers, although in each there is evidence of language impairment at specific language layers. Karen's signing shows many *literal* paraphasias (sublexical substitutions of parameters for intended signs); yet her sentences are grammatically complete and fluent; she uses appropriately and consistently the spatial syntactic mechanisms of the language (the means by which signs are related to one another in sentences, such as verb indexing, index shifting, maintaining coreferentiality). However, she tends not to specify the nominals associated with her spatial indices. In conversation, the examiner always had to ask who or what was the topic of her syntactically correct descriptions. The other patient, Paul, produces a wide array of primarily *grammmatical* paraphasias. He has a proliferation of nouns—but tends to avoid spatial indexing. Paul uses the spatial syntactic mechanisms of the language sparsely, and when he does, he typically fails to specify the spatial relations between signs correctly (see figure 29A). For example, in signing the ASL equivalent of "We arrived (at a place) and stayed there," the correct adult form would require agreement of spatial loci for ARRIVE, STAY (THERE). Paul instead indexed the signs incorrectly to three different loci.

In this respect, the two fluent patients show markedly different patterns: preservation of the spatially encoded syntactic mechanisms but failure to specify nominals for the indices in Karen's signing; and preservation of lexical items (despite many semantic and morphological errors) but failure in the spatial syntactic underpinnings on the part of Paul.

What is striking about these results is not simply that language functions have been differentially affected in the three left-lesioned signers, but that these patients exhibit dissociations of language components specific to the structure of sign language: agrammatic nonfluent signing in one patient;

fluent signing in two patients, but predominantly literal paraphasias in one and grammatical paraphasias in the other.

The dissociation evident in Paul's language breakdown is
of particular interest; there appears to be a separation between
sign-based morphology and syntax-based morphology. Paul
fails to use (or uses indifferently) inflections for person and
number in his signing, and these, together with the system
of indexic reference, form part of the syntactic underpinnings
of sentence structure in ASL. However, Paul's signing is
nonetheless fluent and not lacking in other aspects of morphology. There are pervasive paragrammaticisms in his
signing: semantic and morphological substitutions and even
morphological augmentations. (Figure 29B gives a few
examples.)

It is of considerable potential significance that there is
great similarity in the kinds of errors Paul makes in both
ASL and written English. Shortly after his stroke, Paul wrote,

I spoke to the axiom in the window. I sprintered the Green
aside the window. Many times as I looked at the Capitol I
wonder the many times were engaged at the same time by
the representatives as they behaved the problems."

While not complete jargon, this poststroke writing is typical
of hearing Wernicke's patients. There are semantic misuses
as well as neologisms, yet there are long syntactically correct
sequences.

Remarkably, Paul's ASL signing exhibits these same properties: relatively fluent long stretches of sign, some aspects
of complex structure, but many semantic misuses and even
certain unwarranted inflections. Paul's consistent tendency
in ASL, in addition to this, is to elaborate—to interject a
morphologically complex sign where an uninflected one
would have been appropriate. He uses and augments inflections for temporal aspect, manner, degree, and derivational processes. However, Paul fails to use, or consistently
misuses, certain other ASL inflections—for person, reciprocity, and number. He is, in fact, deficient specifically in

those inflectional processes in ASL that are intimately bound up with specifying the relations between signs in a sentence, that is, those inflectional processes that, together with indexing, provide the grammatical scaffolding of ASL sentence grammar. And, significantly, these are precisely the processes that involve the manipulation of space in signing (Padden, Bellugi, and Poizner, 1982).

From these studies of left-hemisphere-damaged deaf patients, we find that different structural layers of signed language can be selectively impaired by neurological damage. Furthermore, we find strikingly that in some patients there can be a complete separation for linguistic and visual-spatial capacities, even in a visual-spatial language. By looking at a language with a radically different input-output system, we seek to provide a unique perspective on the relation between language-specific and channel-specific neural mechanisms and, at the same time, confront fundamental issues concerning brain plasticity.

Acknowledgments

This work was supported in part by National Science Foundation grant #BNS81–11479 and National Institutes of Health grant #NS15175 and HD13249 to The Salk Institute for Biological Studies. Illustrations were drawn by Frank A. Paul and are copyright © 1983 by Ursula Bellugi.

Notes

1. *Notation Conventions*: Words in capital letters refer to English glosses for ASL signs. The gloss represents the meaning of the unmodulated basic form of a sign. A bracketed superscript following a sign gloss indicates that the sign is made with some regular change in form associated with a systematic change in meaning and thus indicates grammatical operations on signs. Either the inflection or the meaning can be specified. Points in space associated with indexing are marked by subscripted location indices (i, j), indicating

agreement markers, and person reference is indicated by subscripted ·
numerals (for example, 3 indicates 3rd person). Inflectional forms
embedded within other inflections are indicated by nested brackets.

Comments

If the notion of language as a biologically autonomous system,
itself composed of autonomous subsystems or modules, is
to be sustained, it is crucial that some degree of correspondence be established between the structures of signed and
spoken languages. A striking divergence between the two
modes (if we may accept ASL as a prototypical signed language) appears in the relation between the formational (phonological) systems deployed for lexical and grammatical, or
syntactical, purposes. In spoken languages these systems are
identical; the set of phonemes used for grammatical distinctions is a subset of those used for lexical distinctions
(thus /s/ serves to distinguish both *cats* from *cat* and *base*
from *bay*). By contrast, in ASL movements of the hand used
for grammatical distinctions are quite different from those
used for lexical distinctions; in fact, ASL syntax may even
draw from a class of movements not available to the lexicon
at all, namely, those of the face rather than the hand. This
difference between the two types of language seems to stem
from their difference in modality. While a language addressed
to the ear can rely on *sequential* structure and may therefore
use the same set of phonemic elements in a different order
to convey a particular morphemic distinction, a signed language, addressing a more or less *simultaneous* nest of gestures
to the eye, must make the components of the pattern formally
distinct. Thus ASL provides an explicit surface distinction
between lexicon and syntax that is altogether absent from
spoken languages.

This difference between the two modes of language raises
a question about their underlying relation. Is signed language
merely an analog, or is it a true homolog of spoken language?

Do the two modes share nothing but function, like the wing of a bird and the wing of a bat? Or do they also share some underlying structural origin, a common base of syntactic or motoric control that emerges in two functionally equivalent, but diverse, forms?

The answer may come from a comparison of aphasic deficits in the two languages. The case studies reported by Bellugi provide persuasive evidence that the left hemisphere is crucially involved in the *production* of signed no less than spoken language. Moreover, the modes of breakdown are not simply motoric, but are remarkably analogous to the fluent and nonfluent modes of spoken-language breakdown, while yet reflecting patterns unique to sign. We thus have preliminary evidence for a shared neurological base in the output of the two languages. Should we therefore expect to find also a left-hemisphere perceptuomotor link in sign?

Here the effects of right-hemisphere lesions will be of particular interest. In spoken language right-hemisphere damage is associated with "dysprosody," that is, monotonic speech (although no one, it seems, has tested for the double dissociation that we might reasonably predict between affective and syntactic functions of prosody due to right and left lesions). But it is not clear what effect, if any, we should expect a right-hemisphere lesion to have on sign language. Should the reliance on visuospatial structure yield perceptual deficits? Or is it implausible that perception and production are controlled from opposite hemispheres? Are there analogies between aspects of sign modulation and spoken intonation that would lead us to expect sign "dysprosody"? Whatever the answers, comparative studies of the neurological bases of spoken and signed aphasia should bear decisively on our view of their relation as one of analogy or homology.

Syntactic Competence in Agrammatism — A Lexical Hypothesis

D. Caplan

This paper presents a hypothesis concerning the nature of what may be called "grammatical competence" in agrammatic patients. The hypothesis seeks to reconcile some apparently conflicting empirical observations of the abilities of agrammatic patients to interpret sentences in tasks of auditory comprehension. The paper does not attempt to prove the hypothesis, but does indicate various types of sentential material relevant to a test of its validity. The hypothesis constitutes a specific suggestion concerning linguistic theories of agrammatism. There is a link between any such theory and theories of language structure itself: The optimal linguistic analysis of agrammatism may be more compatible with some particular view of language structures and their processing than with some other view. If it can be shown that agrammatism is not the result of some new brain function and if the reliability of the particular analysis of agrammatism (that is, the reliability of data collection, the generalization of observations to at least one well-defined subset of agrammatic patients, and so on) is demonstrated, then agrammatism—like any other aphasic syndrome or symptom meeting these conditions—would help choose between linguistic theories. There has been a number of suggestions along these lines in the recent literature, including some work on agrammatism (Bradley, Garrett, and Zurif, 1980) that, in my opinion, deserves careful attention from linguists and psycholinguists.

Nonetheless, I shall have little to say about this issue, given the quite speculative nature of the hypothesis presented here.

Empirical studies of the performance of agrammatic patients, in tasks other than speech production, have demonstrated that these patients have previously unsuspected difficulties with these tasks. Goodglass and his coworkers (Goodglass et al., 1979) showed that Broca's aphasics have less difficulty understanding conjoined sentences than sentences expressing identical propositional content by means of reduced relative clauses. Heilman and Scholes (1978) demonstrated a lack of sensitivity in Broca's aphasics to the disambiguation of indirect objects in sentences such as

1. John showed her baby pictures.

when disambiguation is accomplished by insertion of the definite article before *baby* or before *pictures*. Zurif and Caramazza (1976) showed that agrammatic patients cannot choose between correct and incorrect depictions of the relations between nouns, verbs, and adjectives in sentences with center-embedded, semantically reversible relative clauses, but that they can do so with identical syntactic material that is not semantically reversible; moreover, they systematically misinterpret syntactically identical material that is semantically improbable. Saffran, Schwartz, and Marin (1980) reported that agrammatic patients cannot appreciate functional relations determined by word order in reversible active and passive sentences, both when the subject matter is unrelated to events in the real world and when it is so related but is semantically reversible.

Zurif and Caramazza (1976) interpreted their observations as reflecting an inability of agrammatic patients to process sentence form in an "algorithmic" fashion. In their view, agrammatic patients use "heuristic strategies" by which the lexical semantic content of nouns, verbs, and adjectives is accessed and integrated, without benefit of syntax, into semantic/conceptual structures relating the semantic content to possible or probable events in the real world. Thus, in their view, agrammatic patients do not construct syntactic representations, and their failure to do so reflects a more fundamental disorder in the use of closed-class/function words, at least under real time-processing conditions. Saffran, Schwartz, and Marin (1980) suggested a somewhat different interpretation of their own data. According to these authors, the agrammatic patient cannot represent functional relations of nouns around verbs, in a Fillmore (1968) case grammar; this leads to an inability to use information derived from word order in the comprehension of sentences. Berndt and Caramazza (1980) hypothesized that errors elicited from agrammatic subjects in a large variety of tests can be attributed to a failure of the human parser, conceived as constructed along the lines suggested by Kimball (1973).

All three views propose a strong hypothesis, linking disturbances in different modalities, in such a way that there is a (roughly) parallel disturbance in both speech production and speech comprehension. The disturbance, extending in some studies to other psycholinguistic modalities of language use, is said to be explained by the "central" nature of the processing deficit. Goodglass (1980) has questioned this interpretation on the grounds that strict parallelism between performance on input and output tasks has never been demonstrated in individual patients. The doubts expressed by Goodglass can reasonably be extended to ask whether individual groups of agrammatic subjects, described in the literature, would each have behaved as the others did on the still few comprehension tasks on which they have been tested.

Moreover, quite apart from these justifiable doubts, certain data in the recent literature are hard to reconcile with the hypotheses stated. At least three papers indicate that agrammatic (or Broca's) aphasics *can* use some syntactic structures in a receptive language task. Andreewski and Seron (1975) studied a single agrammatic patient's ability to read words, such as *car* in French, that are category-ambiguous between an open-class item and a closed-class item. The words were read successfully regardless of whether they were embedded in lists containing only open-class or only closed-class items, and a number of semantic paraphasias were produced relating only to the open-class meaning of the words presented. Moreover, this patient was able to read the homonym as an open-class word in a sentence, but not as a closed-class word, even in cases where the two homophonic forms were used in the same sentence. Andreeski and Seron argue that this behavior—admittedly not a direct test of comprehension—indicated sensitivity to category information and the ability of the patient to recover categorial labels from sentential information. Lineberger, Schwartz, and Saffran (1981) presented data indicating that one agrammatic patient, who performed at chance levels on the passive test of Saffran, Schwartz, and Marin, could detect a wide variety of grammatical errors in sentences on a grammatical judgment task.

Caplan, Matthei, and Gigley (1981) investigated the ability of a group of eleven Broca's aphasics (not all agrammatic) to understand functional relations around gerunds in English. The sentences are

2. Can you show John fighting the soldiers?

3. Can you show John the fighting soldiers?

4. Can you show John the fighting of the soldiers?

5. Can you show John bravely fighting the soldiers?

6. Can you show John the brave fighting of the soldiers?

Possible functional relations are determined by the location of the definite article. In a play task involving manipulation of objects, a subgroup of five Broca's aphasics showed near-perfect sensitivity to the location of the definite article as a determinant of possible functional relations of the post-matrix-verb noun phrase and the gerund, while a second group of patients did not show this sensitivity. The first group was also clearly sensitive to differences between participial and nominative gerundive forms. The group of five patients who were not sensitive to restrictions on using the post-matrix-verb noun phrase as subject of the nominative gerund, marked by the position of the definite article, nonetheless had no tendency to use the postgerundive noun phrase as subject of the gerund, even in semantically reversible conditions. In other words, one group of Broca's aphasics appreciated normal syntactic "control" features of noun phrases marked by the definite article; and a second (possibly more impaired) group demonstrated a strong reliance on the linear order of noun phrases around gerunds, in the assignment of functional relations.

Assume for the moment that these results can be generalized to the broader population of agrammatic subjects. Is it then possible to reconcile the claims of the investigators cited with the apparent discrepancies in the use of the definite article to signify syntactic structure in the material of Caplan et al. versus that of Heilman and Scholes and also with the apparent sensitivity of Andreeski and Seron's patient to syntactic category of homophones in sentential context? The hypothesis I shall present attempts to account for these apparently discrepant observations. I shall call this hypothesis the "lexical node hypothesis." According to this hypothesis, agrammatic patients do achieve a certain degree of syntactic representation in sentence comprehension, and probably in production as well. The syntactic representation available to these patients, according to the lexical-node hypothesis, is lexical category information of open-class items, that is, the syntactic labels N, V, A (noun, verb, adjective).

This information is available from two sources. The first may be considered "bottom-up." This source is lexical identification itself. In all cases, agrammatic aphasics have access to the lexicon, and, by hypothesis, in the case of nouns, verbs, and adjectives, the lexical representations that they access include lexical category information. This information is sometimes unambiguous, but in most cases, of course, category ambiguities cannot be resolved by lexical identity and must be disambiguated by syntactic structures in sentence context. I shall return to the issue of this sentential disambiguation.

Pursuing for the moment the question of lexical information available to agrammatic subjects, we may speculate as to whether the lexicon itself provides any further structural information for these patients. That sentences are interpreted at all and that open-class vocabulary items are grouped according to what may, very roughly, be termed thematic relations in the so-called metalinguistic judgment tasks reported by Zurif, Caramazza, and Myerson (1972) and by Kolk (1978), as well as evidence from certain aspects of F_0 contours in agrammatic subjects (Cooper, 1980), suggest that some supralexical structure is available to these patients. Is it syntactic, semantic, or pragmatic?

One possibility consistent with the lexical node hypothesis is that syntactic information, lexically arrayed against open-class items, can be accessed by agrammatic patients. There are some natural candidates for what this information might be—at least in some versions of lexical theory, such as that represented in Chomsky (1965). I would like to propose that syntactic representations associated with each open-class lexical item are subcategorization frames (Chomsky, 1965). (I shall return to issues raised by expanded lexical structures.)

An alternative to the notion that syntactic information of this kind is available to agrammatic patients would be that the organizing principles relating words on the tasks cited are semantic or pragmatic. To distinguish between these two possibilities it would be relevant to investigate strict subcategorization features of verbs that are not semantically determined. Thus sentences such as

7. John put the bicycle in the garage.

can be contrasted with

8. John pushed the bicycle in the garage.

Put but not *pushed* is obligatorily subcategorized for a locative phrase, and sequences such as

9. John put the bicycle.

are unacceptable, while sentences such as

10. John pushed the bicycle.

are acceptable. The syntactic nature of subcategorization information seems unequivocal in these cases, and differential appreciation of the relation between locative phrases and the verb, as could be demonstrated on a variety of experimental tasks, would be relevant.

One consequence of the speculation that agrammatic aphasics may have access to lexical subcategorization features of the open-class vocabulary is that, by this means, they may have at their disposal a variety of supralexical category node labels not available through representation of phrase structures derived from the base and transformational components of a grammar. That is to say, the lexical representations accessed through lexical identification of the open-class vocabularies may include syntactic structures that use nodes such as PP, NP, VP, S, S̄, and other supralexical category nodes.

One way of ascertaining whether agrammatic patients, if they are sensitive at all to the existence of supralexical category nodes, are aware of these nodes by virtue of lexical rather than phrase structure knowledge would be to contrast sentences in which these nodes (and other features of sentence structure) are (at least partially) lexically determined with others in which they are not. Thus, for instance, sentences such as

11. John promised Bill to see a doctor.

12. John persuaded Bill to see a doctor.

can be contrasted with relative-clause structures. In both cases, there are embedded sentences present; but in sentences 11 and 12, embedded sentences are mentioned in the subcategorization features of the matrix verb, which also determines the identity of the superficially absent subject-noun phrase in the embedded sentence. One would expect, by this

hypothesis, that agrammatic patients would show appreciation of this aspect of the structure of these sentences, in
contrast to their apparent difficulties in understanding the
functional relations around embedded verbs in relative
clauses, which are not lexically marked.

Moving from these speculations regarding the consequnces
of accessing lexically determined syntactic information to
the issue of disambiguating category-ambiguous open-class
items, we note a variety of structural elements that serve to
disambiguate such items in sentences.

The first such element is clearly the closed-class vocabulary. One way to reconcile the apparent discrepancy between
the results of Heilman and Scholes's experiment and the
performance of one subgroup of patients in the work of
Caplan et al. with gerundive constructions is to note that in
the indirect-object constructions, lexical categories do not
change as a result of the disambiguation imposed by the
position of the definite article. In both forms of the indirect
object, the lexical category immediately dominating the individual words is N (noun). The position of the definite
article determines whether the supralexical category that
dominates the N is an NP or another N. This is precisely
the kind of information that the lexical node hypothesis states
is unavailable to agrammatic patients, unless by virtue of
subcategorization features of the open-class vocabulary. In
the gerundive constructions, the location of the definite article
also determines where the category N is to be assigned; however, in the case where the definite article follows the gerund,
the lexical category that dominates the gerund is V rather
than N. If we hypothesize that the role of the closed-class
vocabulary is restricted to disambiguating different lexical
categories and does not involve the assignment of supralexical
categories, the difference between these two sets of experimental materials would naturally follow.

A number of predictions regarding the ability of agrammatic patients to distinguish certain sentence forms and not

others naturally follow from this hypothesis. One would expect, for instance, that the contrast between the perfect and passive participles in sentences such as

13. Has the dog eaten the bone?

14. Has the dog the eaten bone?

(not the most felicitous examples) would be appreciated because of the category change from verb to adjective. Similarly, the verb-adjective change in the following two sentences ought to lead to an appreciation of the relation between *man* and *fried*:

15. Can you show that the man fried the fish?

16. Can you show the man the fried fish?

Similarly, the noun-verb differences in the following sentences ought to be appreciated and influence the relation between *man* and *catch*:

17. Can you show the man catch the fish?

18. Can you show the man the catch of fish?

On the other hand, it would be expected that compound nouns that are not lexicalized, and that consist of N-N sequences, such as the term *baby pictures* used in the experiments of Heilman and Scholes, could not be assigned a compound-noun category feature. Verbal compounds such as a *man-eating shark* would similarly not be ambiguous and would be indistinguishable from sequences such as *the man eating the shark*. (Both these cases presume that lexical transformational rules of word formation are not available to the agrammatic patient, that is, that only subcategorization features are accessed in his lexicon.)

The lexical-node hypothesis provides several parameters along which one can look for possible recovery and variation in agrammatism. It is conceivable that, as agrammatic patients improve, one feature of the linguistic structures they reacquire is supralexical category nodes introduced by phrase structure and transformation rules. If this is the case, we may consider the further possibility that supralexical nodes are reintroduced into grammatical analyses of these patients in accordance with a "depth" analysis by which the first nonlexical category nodes to be recovered are those immediately dominating lexical category nodes; more deeply embedded structures would only reemerge or be reacquired later, in proportion to their nodal distances from lexical category nodes. Quite a number of specific hypotheses can be entertained within this framework.

Two final issues arise with respect to the lexical-node hypothesis. The first is the relation of this hypothesis, stated before in terms of an *Aspects* theory of lexical structure, to the possibility that lexical structures are significantly richer than those of Chomsky (1965). What if lexical structures are as rich in syntactic information as postulated by Bresnan (1980), Wasow (1977), and others? The lexical-node hypothesis is, of course, compatible with an enriched lexicon; but if syntactic information, represented lexically for each open-class vocabulary item was indeed sufficient for the construction of complex phrase markers, the consequences of a syntactic competence restricted to purely lexical syntactic information would be much less severe than if the lexical structures were relatively impoverished. Even with an enriched lexicon, one would expect to find that some syntactic structures are not available to agrammatic aphasics; moreover, several aspects of the interpretation of "logical form" (Chomsky, 1980) over syntactic structures would still be expected to be unavailable to agrammatics. More significantly, however, the possibility of an enriched lexicon suggests that we look for taxonomies of lexical processes. It is obviously premature to claim that we could choose between theories of lexical processes on the basis of their compatibility with agrammatic performance; but it seems to me that if analysis of agrammatism strongly supports a particular view of the syntactic information available to a well-defined group of patients and if this view is more easily expressed within one particular account of the lexicon, then this constitutes evidence, of the sort alluded to initially in this chapter, in favor of one particular linguistic analysis.

The second and final issue is that among the "top-down" or "sentential" cues for disambiguation of lexical category nodes, when lexical items are themselves category ambiguous, there are likely to be other features of sentential form, in addition to the syntactic consequences of the closed-class vocabulary. For example, we might expect a variety of intonational cues to be pertinent at this level. It might then be that certain subgroups of aphasics, including subgroups of agrammatic aphasics, are sensitive to certain classes of cues, such as those carried by intonation, but not to certain others, such as the consequences of the closed-class vocabulary.

In summary, I have presented one hypothesis suggested to me by several recent results regarding agrammatism. It seems to me that as Kean (1980) has pointed out, we are at a stage in "linguistic aphasiology" where the statement of hypotheses at this level of detail is possible—and indeed a useful guide to research.

Aspects of Sentence Processing in Aphasia

E. B. Zurif

There are two related questions that I want to address very briefly. First, are there underlying uniformities in the ways in which focal brain damage exerts its effects on the separate activities of speaking and listening? Second, if there are important overarching constraints, can they be interpreted in terms of modern psycholinguistic concepts? Recent analyses of Broca's aphasia incline me toward supposing that there are positive answers to both questions.

The work I have in mind has been concerned with explaining the dissociation between, on the one hand, the telegraphic output and otherwise syntactically impoverished speech in Broca's aphasia and, on the other hand, the clinical impression of their relatively intact comprehension. The approach taken in this work, typically, has been to probe the less public comprehension capacities of these patients, mostly by the use of sentence-picture matching paradigms. And the general finding is that their comprehension is abnormally dependent upon semantic and contextual constraints (for reviews see Berndt and Caramazza, 1980, 1981). Specifically, for sentences more complicated than simple actives (though here, too, there is some doubt), Broca's aphasic patients seem to rely on the referential values of individual words and plausibility constraints—that is, they appear to sample from among the content words and to combine their meanings in terms of what they know about the world. When such constraints are absent—when it "makes sense," for example, for either of two noun phrases in a passive sentence to serve as agent—their comprehension fails (see, for example, Caramazza and Zurif, 1976).

In effect, then, comprehension and production skills are not so readily separated by anterior brain damage as clinical impression would have it. But more than this: It has seemed to a number of us that this overarching limitation may be interpreted as the consequence of a disruption to a central, and language-specific, component—more particularly, to a device geared to syntactic analyses for all language activities (Zurif and Blumstein, 1978; for reading see Samuels and Benson, 1979; for writing see Goodglass and Hunter, 1970).

Having entered this generalization, it must now be tempered. Thus Goodglass (1980; and see his chapters in parts I and III) has noted that the evidence for a strict parallel between production and comprehension limitations has not yet been established on an individual patient basis. Some efforts have been made in this respect (Caramazza et al., 1981; Schwartz, Saffran, and Marin, 1980; Saffran, Schwartz, and Marin, 1980), but until now the notion of a neurologically isolable syntactic component has been developed largely on the basis of statistical inference. And the generalization does not transparently apply to all patients with agrammatic output. There exist a number of reports—graced by careful testing—of patients who have shown structural abnormalities in their output, who yet show what seems to be a normal ability to comprehend (see, for example, Kolk, 1981; Miceli et al., 1981). Possibly, as neurological assessment techniques are further refined, these behavioral exceptions will be shown to correspond to exceptions at the neurological level and thereby to index finer-grained distinctions at this latter level.

Admittedly, it could turn out to be otherwise. Comprehension and production are, after all, very different activities. Thus while comprehension systems, as Garrett (1981) puts it, "can play fast and loose with sentence form so long as interpretation survives," production processes must be precisely responsive to grammatical form if the speaker is not to sound funny. It may be, therefore, that the processes of comprehension are heavily contextually grounded, whereas, in apparent contrast, production processes are more intimately linked to syntactic levels of representation.

In this context, then, although comprehension and production deficits usually cooccur in agrammatic aphasia, and although both seem to limit syntactic processing, these may yet be differently based and thereby dissociable—in principle, and at times, even in practice. I expect, however, that this supposed dissociation will prove incorrect. In fact, there are even now some indications that it is incorrect and that we might more profitably pursue the notion of an overarching selective impairment in syntactic processing.

The evidence—such as it is—implicates processes involving the use of closed-class items. Specifically, just as these patients on clinical observation tend to omit grammatical morphemes in their output, so too do they seem to be unable to use such items as structural markers when listening to sentences and in other receptive and metalinguistic tasks. This less clinically obvious point has emerged from studies using a range of paradigms: relatedness judgments (see, for example, Zurif and Caramazza, 1976); anagram tasks (von Stockert and Bader, 1976); lexical decision tasks (Bradley, Garrett, and Zurif, 1980); a letter-cross-out method (Rosenberg et al., 1982); and a word-monitoring task that may be considered as tapping on-line processing (Swinney, Zurif, and Cutler, 1980). With the exception of the cross-out experiment, all of the findings gained from these studies have been duly reported in the literature; for present purposes, I want to excerpt only a very few of these findings.

The relatedness judgment task (Zurif and Caramazza, 1976)—though flawed by virtue of unspecifiable "demand" variables—is nonetheless noteworthy for the evidence it raises concerning the distinction between the syntactic role of function words and their semantic or "functional" force. Thus when patients were asked to judge how written words in a sentence "go best together," they generally failed to integrate the function words of the sentence. As a consequence, their judgments violated the integrity of phrasal constituents. There was one exception to this general finding, however; this involved prepositions, and then only when they were clearly and nonredundantly "functional"—containing, for example, important locative information. In such situations, agrammatic aphasic patients consistently clustered the prepositions with the relevant nouns.

Later work by Friederici (1982) has confirmed this pattern; using a fill-in-the-blank task, she has observed that Broca's aphasics are significantly more likely to produce prepositions that have obvious semantic content than those that are only syntactically relevant.

In effect, in controlled experimental tasks, Broca's aphasics seem better able to produce and acknowledge the existence of prepositions that fix the functional relations of nouns to verbs than they do function words that serve as syntactic placeholders. Possibly, this reflects a neurologically honored distinction between representational levels, by which the implementation of semantically interpretable relations contacts one neurological level, and processes involving function words in the surface assignment of phrasal constituents contacts another (Garrett, 1982). Prepositions could be involved at both levels, depending upon the sentential context, and therefore be relatively impervious to the effects of left anterior brain damage.

Clearly, these remarks constitute a preliminary and imprecise characterization of the Broca's syntactic problem. Indeed, it may well be that the contrast between the processing of sentence form and that of sentence meaning should not be cast in terms of the partition between function and content words. Syntactic processes involving function words may be only one of the structure-building operations affected by left anterior brain damage, or even only a reflection of a larger problem. We still do not know, for example, whether when Broca's aphasics use verbs they are actually using them to predicate or merely as labels of actions. The relevant experiments remain to be done.

A final comment: While my remarks to this point have had to do with the effects of damage to left anterior cortex, they should not be construed as suggesting that it is *only* this area of cortex upon which syntactic processing can be so precisely delimited. Wernicke's aphasic patients also seem to have syntactic problems; and so the question arises, is syntax a "weak link"—the most vulnerable to brain damage, wherever its site? We cannot, at present, rule out this possibility. However, I think that it is rather uninteresting to root it to demonstrations that Broca's and Wernicke's aphasics are similar insofar as they are both less likely to comprehend sentences that are "more difficult" than those that are "less difficult" (see, for example, Boller, Kim, and Mack, 1977)—the metric for difficulty presumably resting on the fact that normals find some constructions more difficult than others. Comprehension failures can stem from very different causes; and in fact, if one looks closely, Broca's and Wernicke's aphasics do show some differences in their comprehension breakdowns (see, for example, Caramazza and Zurif, 1976).

To be sure, the interpretation of these differences remains elusive and will require confronting the likelihood that there exist a number of distinct levels of syntactic processing. But possibly the clinically contrasting syndromes of Broca's and Wernicke's aphasias will serve to disentangle these levels.

Acknowledgment

Some of the work reported here was supported by NIH grants 11408, 15972, and 06209.

Comments

Caplan's lexical node hypothesis does not reject the notion of a single, central representation of syntax, as proposed by Zurif. On the contrary, Caplan effectively undertakes to defend this notion by attempting to reconcile apparent discrepancies in the reported syntactic capacities of agrammatic patients. He proposes to do this by acknowledging sources of syntactic information other than word order and closed-class/function words, and he makes an ingenious and explicit hypothesis as to one possible source.

The discussion that followed Caplan's and Zurif's presentations skirted the somewhat technical, linguistic issues Caplan had raised and concentrated on questioning the notion of a single, central representation of syntax by pointing to the rarity of parallel input and output deficits. It was argued that many of the claims for comprehension deficits are of dubious value because studies of agrammatic aphasics lack controls. In point of fact, most aphasics, agrammatic or not, fail tests for comprehension of closed-class words.

Moreover, there are ample reports in the older literature (see, for example, Pick, 1913; Oubredane, 1951; Tissot, Mourin and Lhermitte, 1973; Luria, 1947, 1976) of patients who were either receptively, but not expressively, agrammatic or vice versa. It is true that these works often do not supply enough detail to resolve current controversies, but there is also current evidence to support them. Geschwind noted, for example, that it is extremely common for a conduction aphasic to display agrammatic repetition, but grammatical spontaneous speech. He described an aphasic with a subcortical lesion whom he had seen recently, who had slow, but grammatical speech, yet profound difficulty in understanding syntactic distinctions conveyed by closed-class items (for example, "point to the pencil with the fork," "point to the pencil and the fork").

Goodglass followed this up by recalling an early study of his own, testing a patient's ability to detect omission of the -S morpheme of English possessives and plurals; there was no correlation between the patient's ability to produce and his ability to detect omission of the morpheme. Moreover, agrammatic output does not always indicate a central deficit, but may simply arise from a production difficulty. An example comes from a patient who omitted "if" and "it" in trying to repeat the phrase, "If it rains . . . ," but wrote "if" with his finger to indicate that he knew he was supposed to say the word, but could not.

While all these criticisms are well taken, they certainly do not demonstrate that there is no central representation of syntax. Thus the cases of the conduction aphasics may seem to imply double representation of some classes of vocabulary—one for repetition, one for production— but they are also compatible with the notion of a single representation, accessed by different routes in spontaneous speech and in repetition. In any event, as Zurif remarked, there are surely many different levels of possible deficit. Given the theoretical interest of a central syntactic impairment and its direct bearing on the modularity issue, the search for fully parallel agrammatic deficits in input and output should be pursued.

Syntax in Brain-Injured Children   M. Dennis

The independence of syntax from other aspects of language is a central theme of this book. If one accepts that data from brain-injured individuals are relevant to this issue, it is important to ascertain what the relation between data and theory should be and, also, what form the data should take. Generally, theory has preceded data in this area, with particular theoretical positions prompting the search for test data to confirm or disconfirm them. I think this emphasis has been misplaced. It seems to me that theories about the independence of syntax are premature until it can be established from the effects of brain damage that syntax is dissociable from other constituents of language, and so warrants a distinct theoretical treatment.

It is not clear what has been established about syntax from studies of brain injury conducted to date. Although a body of information exists on how aphasics use and understand syntax, broad-spectrum tests of syntax and other language skills in the same individuals are lacking. Tests of particular theories have generally been conducted with diverse groups of patients. Aphasics have been selected for study primarily because of aberrant language behavior, and only incidentally because of their brain injuries; in consequence, it is unclear how syntactic competence varies with different forms, etiologies, and parameters of brain insult. The studies to date have concerned adult aphasic dissolution almost exclusively, with little attention given to anomalous or truncated acquisition. This preoccupation with the adult brain has meant, further, an overrepresentation in the literature of particular forms of cerebral injury (specifically, space-occupying or discharging lesions as opposed to static but anomalous perturbations of brain development). At best, then, studies of the effect of brain injury on syntax have so far provided an incomplete data base from which to consider the question of syntactic independence.

What we need are comprehensive studies of syntax in brain-damaged groups with defined cerebral pathology. Such studies would be directed toward specifying how syntax meshes with the rest of language, that is, how it is correlated with some language functions but dissociated from others. Information of this kind is a necessary prelude to any statement about whether syntax ought to be considered as representationally coherent or logically independent in any theory about language.

Within this framework, I want to discuss three things: first, how syntax fits into the broader language picture in a group of individuals who sustained early brain damage but who are now not so much brain-injured as operating with an atypical language substrate; second, whether the status of syntax within the language system in these individuals is peculiar or whether it has any degree of generality in a larger group of brain-injured children; and third, what such information may suggest, not about the formal features of any neurolinguistic theory of syntax, but about the functional correlations and dissociations any theory will have to explain if it is to account for syntactic development under particular conditions of brain damage.

What of the functional development of syntax in individuals with one hemisphere removed in infancy or childhood? This condition of extreme lateralized cerebral insult early in life requires that language be acquired with only half the normal cortical mass—the typical half, the left hemisphere, or the atypical half, the right hemisphere. The syntax that develops in an early-isolated right hemisphere is poor in both capacity and strategy. If the left hemisphere is removed in infancy or childhood, syntactic comprehension develops slowly (Dennis and Whitaker, 1976) and poorly (Dennis and Kohn, 1975). In relation to the left, the right hemisphere is deficient in using higher-order grammatical structures and syntax-signaling functors (Dennis, 1980a,b). The isolated right hemisphere has a different, more limited, and less efficient set of strategies than the left for understanding syntactically diverse sentences (Dennis, 1980a). The syntactic comprehension of patients with delimited left-hemisphere removals and right-hemisphere speech varies with some aspect of left-hemisphere integrity—structural, functional, or both (Kohn, 1980).

The syntactic deficits of the early-isolated right hemisphere are not exclusively auditory. When the right hemisphere reads, for example, written grammar is not exploited to achieve accuracy and fluency, nor are the higher-order syntactic structures that carry text meaning (Dennis, Lovett, and Wiegel-Crump, 1981).

Having demonstrated a broadly based deficit of syntactic development in the isolated right hemispheres of the hemidecorticate group, we need to consider how syntax relates to the other constituents of language in these individuals. Here one finds a complex pattern.

Syntactic impairments in the isolated right hemispheres are independent of verbal intelligence (Dennis and Kohn, 1975; Kohn, 1980) and also of a wide variety of phonological and lexical semantic functions: articulation; auditory discrimination; letter- and word-category fluency; single-word comprehension; lexical retrieval to semantic or visual cues; and the comprehension of canonical sentences (Dennis and Kohn, 1975; Dennis and Whitaker, 1976; Dennis, 1980b).

Aspects of sentence meaning that are carried by particular syntactic forms are, as might be expected, relatively inaccessible to the isolated right hemispheres. Although these individuals identify the lexical semantics of a sentence, they generally ignore thematic information about subject and topic because such information is conveyed by variations in syntactic structure like the passive, cleft, and pseudocleft sentence forms (Dennis, 1980b).

Those language systems that share certain features with syntax—notably a quasi-formal or rule-governed structure—seem to break down or to be poorly developed in right-hemisphere individuals with poor syntax. For example, the ability to infer a morphophonemic rule from experience with written English and to apply it to the reading of nonsense words is less efficient in the right than in the left isolated hemisphere (Dennis, Lovett, and Wiegel-Crump, 1981). Perhaps more dramatic is the distinction between real-world knowledge about a word and the syntactic computations the word enters into. Each isolated hemisphere can establish the premise of verbs like *remember*, but the right is inaccurate at determining the implications of the same word in the same sentence because the latter ability depends on the interaction of verb type with sentence surface structure syntax. In general, language tasks that require the deployment of stored knowledge about words or sentences seem within the capacity of either isolated hemisphere; the right is deficient when active computation and rule use are critical to establishing meaning.

The longer the utterance to be used or understood, the more likely it is that active linguistic computation will be needed. One would expect, then, that the isolated right hemisphere would have difficulty in extracting the full meaning of higher-order language constituents like texts and stories, despite its demonstrated ability to derive meaning from single words and simple sentences. Indeed, this seems to be the case. The syntax of ideas as expressed in texts and stories is less well articulated in the right hemisphere than in the left. In retelling simple stories, the right hemisphere, although fluent, shows a loose rather than tight or embedded episodic structure, a restricted range of connectives linking story propositions, and a redundant rather than efficient system of referential cohesion (Dennis and Lovett, 1982; Dennis, Newman, and Lovett, 1982).

These results show a distinct pattern of correlation and dissociation of function within the language system for individuals with atypical language acquisition substrates. What happens when focal left-hemisphere damage is sustained in later childhood is not fully known, but some evidence suggests that the pattern of syntactic impairment is not the same. If the left hemisphere is damaged by arteritic stroke in later childhood, the child's syntactic deficits are of a different kind, involving morphology as well as the use and understanding of grammar, that is, dysfluency and poor articulation, agrammatism, and a loss of tacit syntactic knowledge (Dennis, 1980c). The manifestation of syntactic defect may change depending on the child's age at time of brain injury and on the type of pathology, although at least two different conditions of left-hemisphere disorder—early hemidecortication and later stroke—can alter syntactic development.

In order to judge the generality of the findings about hemidecorticate syntax in terms of the broader spectrum of brain damage in children, a battery of language tests was administered to a large group ($N=196$) of brain-injured children. The tests sampled many language skills: phonemic discrimination; articulation; word retrieval to semantic, rhyming, and picture cues; fluency to letters and word-category cues; naming prototypicality; combinatorial semantic skills involving integration of verb class with matrix verb and complement negation; comprehension of premise and entailment; judgment of violations in lexical selection, surface structure, and case assignment; comprehension of different syntactic forms whose surface structures are not explicit with respect to underlying grammatical relations; production of tag questions from the surface-structure syntax of heard declaratives.

The children had sustained diverse forms of brain insult with respect to age at onset and at test, to pathology and etiology (congenital malformations; histological anomalies; cerebrovascular accidents; traumata), to location of damage, and to accompanying physical symptoms.

A factor analysis was performed on the children's language tests. Eight factors were needed to account for the variance in test scores, showing that the test battery sampled not one, but a variety of language functions. The syntax tests were separable from the other language measures, in that they were represented principally on three of the eight factors. But the tests were also diverse and varied in terms of their pattern of loading on individual factors. In a large group of brain-injured children, then, variance in syntactic ability can to some extent be separated from other language functions—the children do not pass and fail syntax tests the way they pass or fail any other language test—but there is a degree of diversity within the syntactic function that reflects its interrelations with other constituents of the language system. Under both the special condition of single-hemisphere acquisition and a broad range of brain-damage conditions in childhood, syntax is related to one set of constituents of language but functions quite independently of another. The details of this remain to be specified. It may well be, for example, that the particular pattern of functional development observed in the hemidecorticate group is not identical to that seen in other pathological conditions.

The hemidecorticate studies of syntax, nevertheless, do provide some constraints on theories about the importance of the left hemisphere for early language acquisition. What must be grasped in any such account is not just some general superiority of left hemisphere over right hemisphere (the typical evidence domain of theories in this area), but the particular pattern of correlation and dissociation observed— in effect, how syntax fits into the language system under conditions of anomalous lateralization.

Comments

In subsequent discussion Dennis emphasized the importance of distinguishing among the effects of brain damage incurred at different stages in life and with different etiologies. Time of brain injury is critical. No major reorganization of brain function follows lesions acquired late in life, while substantial reorganization follows lesions *in utero*, with undamaged areas increasing in size and even becoming "supertalented." More subtle changes may follow from postnatal, early childhood lesions of the left hemisphere; language may recover—or, at least, display no obvious deficits—but at the expense of the right hemisphere's normal visuospatial function.

The distinction between anomalous brain organization in the child with congenital abnormalities and lesion effects in a previously intact brain is an important one. But what distinguishes the brain lesion of the child from that of the adult is not just age or time of injury, but pathology. In fact, many of the comparisons between brain injuries in children and brain injuries in adults are based on pathologies so diverse as to be meaningless. The claim that recovery from aphasia is better among children than among adults, for instance, is based largely on comparisons between head injuries in children and strokes in adults. If we compare children and adults with the same pathology, at least some of the behavioral effects may be more similar than has been suspected. A left-hemisphere arteritic stroke in a child produces a reasonably long-term agrammatism that shares at least some features of the adult aphasic stroke patient (Dennis, 1980c).

Before attempting to understand how brain damage affects individuals at different stages in life, one must specify the stage of assessment in relation to the brain insult. In adults the main lesion effect is usually apparent soon after the insult, whereas in children the real consequences of the lesion may not be apparent for many years, until the normal course of cognitive development is completed.

The brain calls on different skills at different stages in development. It is not surprising, therefore, that the picture of lesion effects we draw will vary with the kind of skill considered. For example, the cross-modal associative aspect of reading is probably more important in the early stages of learning to read, while the syntax of texts and sentences becomes significant later, in reading extended prose units. Bearing this in mind, we shall eventually have to explain some of the age-dependent effects of lesions on reading. Why, for example, may loss of the right hemisphere at the age of 6 1/2 prevent a child from learning to read, while loss of the right hemisphere at the age of 30 may have no effect on reading at all? Part of the answer will no doubt involve some subtle interhemispheric facilitation in the acquisition of a complex skill, but another part will probably relate to the kind of reading skills needed at different stages in life.

Finally, the implications of this material for both the localization and the autonomy issues should be noted. Syntax appears to be affected by at least two different anomalies of lateralization, one involving right-hemisphere language acquisition; the other, hemispheric disconnection. While this shows syntax to be lateralized (if not localized), one should not forget that tissue in isolation, deprived of its normal connections, operates differently than it does when it is connected. As far as the autonomy of syntax is concerned, syntax is separable from some aspects of language, but involved in a complex relation to others, such as referential cohesion.

PART V

Prospects for Further   G. A. Ojemann
Brain-Stimulation
Studies during
Neurosurgical
Operations under Local
Anesthesia

This chapter will focus on two questions: How might the techniques of stimulation mapping be used to resolve some of the issues that confront the biologist of language? Do these techniques call our attention to particular issues that have not been raised so far?

Stimulation mapping of the cortex is directed at relating aspects of language behavior and specific cortical areas. There are several advantages to this electrophysiological localization technique: discreteness, reversibility, and the opportunity to observe the effects of stimulation at multiple sites on multiple behaviors. Clear disadvantages include the necessity of using special populations; the unknown physiological mechanism for stimulation effects; and the need to design tests that are repetitive and extremely brief.

An example of the test-construction problem is seen in the phoneme-identification test that has been used in stimulation mapping studies. In this test the subject hears the syllables /aekma/, for example, and during presentation the cortex is stimulated. The subject reports his percept by saying "k" during a time without stimulation that follows the presentation. Of course, this test requires a set of diverse abilities: perception of the syllable, identification of the relevant segment, storage of the percept briefly, and output of the name of the identified item. Since the effects of stimulation end abruptly before the subject emits the overt response, the perceptual test is not confounded by disturbance of response execution. However, further tests must control for the confounding of the other three components of performance. One control has already been tried (Ojemann and Polen, unpublished data); the effect of stimulation on consonant identification (/p,d,g,k/) was compared with that on vowel identification (/i, ʌ/). Identification of stop consonants was impaired at sites where identification of vowels was not. In fact, vowel identification was never disrupted by cortical stimulation. If the cortical disruption were disturbing auditory perception or memory per se, it would likely involve both vowels and consonants.

Data from stimulation mapping studies bear on a number of topics discussed in this book: (1) Can certain language processes be separated neurologically from other language processes and/or from nonlanguage processes? Here, stimulation mapping reveals that a common sensorimotor representation occupies perisylvian sites. These sites seem to be common to the decoding of speech sounds and the generation of orofacial motor outputs especially in sequences (Ojemann and Mateer, 1979a,b; Ojemann, 1980, 1981). (2) Is there a single central representation of the lexicon? There are certainly areas where naming alone is changed by stimulation, and these may play a special role in generating words. The organization of these areas (some found in frontal, some in parietal, some in temporal cortex) might reflect semantic relations or, perhaps, perceptual or response factors. For example, most of the memory effects observed with frontal stimulation are keyed to stimulation during output, while similar effects from parietal and temporal sites are keyed to stimulation at the time of input or during the period when the memory must be stored (Ojemann, 1978; Ojemann and Mateer, 1979a,b; Ojemann, 1980). We might infer, then, that frontal sites related only to naming are involved in retrieval of words during language production, while those in temporal and parietal sites are involved in word storage.

There are also sites where electrically induced changes are confined to closed-class words (Ojemann and Mateer, 1979a; Ojemann, 1980) and where differential roles between frontal and temporal parietal sites might be similar; that is, frontal sites might be involved in retrieval of syntactic forms during language generation, temporal and parietal sites in the storage of these forms. With refined test design these problems of multiple representations in different areas of cortex are amenable to study by stimulation mapping.

There are several issues to which the technique may be extended: How discrete is cortical representation of a language behavior? In a patient whose seizures resulted from disease at age 12 and whose cortex was therefore presumably normal until that age, representation of function was discrete. Adjacent 5-millimeter sites were differentially disruptive in the naming task (Ojemann, 1981). Five millimeters is, of course, gross for the brain (considering the number of neurons involved), and microstimulation with smaller electrodes is clearly the next step in assessing the discreteness of cortical addresses for language functions, that is, for identifying the functional properties of macrocolumns, such as have previously been described in sensory cortices.

How variable are the loci for representation of functions? In the instance of naming, the loci were highly variable over a series of twenty-one patients (Ojemann, 1979, 1981), with the exception of an area anterior to face motor cortex that was rather consistently involved in naming in most subjects. There are far more zones from which naming deficits are produced in males than in females, indicating a potential sexual dimorphism. The chief difference is in frontal naming sites, with few naming failures typically produced by stimulation of anterior frontal sites in females. When changes in naming were evoked in parietal cortex, these tended to be associated with I.Q.s lower than 96, regardless of gender, suggesting a relation between the anatomic substrate of language and overall language abilities. A similar degree of var-

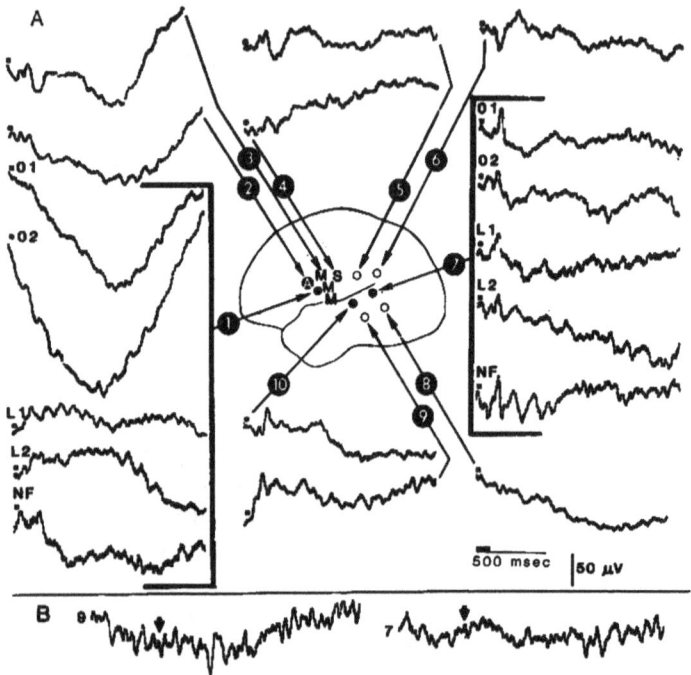

Figure 30.
(*A*) Event-related potentials (ERPs) after 100-msec flashes of O1, the first silently named object picture in name matching, simultaneously recorded from 10 sites in dominant perisylvian cortex of a patient undergoing a craniotomy under local anesthesia. At one posterior site (7) and one premotor site (1), ERPs are also shown for the remaining tasks: O2, L1, L2, and NF. Referential electrocorticogram (ECoG) recordings to linked neck reference were amplified by a 16-channel electroencephalograph (Beckman Acutrace) with bandpass of 0.5–50 Hz. The electrooculogram was recorded from above the right eye. Tracings are average of 34 trials except for NF (17 samples). Only trials free of response errors, eye movements, and other artifacts are averaged. The digitizing rate was 250 samples/sec. Tracings were averaged for 1,500 msec after flash onset (small squares). Positive down. Stimulation mapping of these same cortical sites during naming followed these recordings. Results are indicated on the brain map: M, facial motor cortex; S, sensory cortex; open circles, sites without naming errors; filled circles, sites where stimulation

iability is observed in the location of sites that support reading.

Is the language system rapidly evolving? The variability of functional sites suggests as much (Ojemann, 1979, 1981; Ojemann and Mateer, 1979b), for it underlies verbal skills that have great selective significance. Correlations between level of skills and particular forms of variation associated with the selective pressure would set the stage for rapid evolution of the biologic substrate of language. Some such correlations were observed in the I.Q. study mentioned (Ojemann, 1981).

Which physiological events have anatomic specificity? In other words, can we find electrophysiological correlates specific both to a language behavior and to the particular sites involved in that behavior by stimulation mapping? A first step has been taken in a study employing a silent picture-naming task. The subject sees two pictures, each flashed for 100 milliseconds, separated by 4 to 5 seconds, and then at a cue must report if the names of the depicted items rhyme. Two electrophysiological changes, noted in the electrocor-

---

produced naming errors without arrest of speech (anomia). At sites 1 and 7, anomia was produced on all three trials with stimulation; at site 10, on only 2 or 3 trials. At the site indicated by a circled A, stimulation produced speech arrest on all trials. Error rate on control naming trials without stimulation was zero. Stimulation mapping used 4-msec (peak-to-peak) biphasic pulses, 2.5 msec in total duration, at 60 Hz delivered through electrodes separated by 5 mm. The patient is female and has a verbal I.Q. of 109. Her epileptic focus was confined to the anterior temporal lobe, sparing all ERP recording sites, and was resected after completion of these studies. (B) Single trial recorded simultaneously at sites 7 and 9 for the 500 msec before and 1,500 msec after an O1 object picture was presented (onset indicated by arrow). Calibration is as in (A). In contrast to site 9, note the flattening of the tracing at site 7 beginning with the onset of the flash and the resumption of the high-amplitude oscillations about 900 msec later. (Fried, Ojemann, and Fetz, 1981) ticogram, seem to have both behavioral and anatomical specificity: a slow negative shift in frontal areas and a de-synchronization of activity in posterior areas. The desyn-chronization consists primarily of an attenuation of electrical activity in the 7–12-Hz frequency band; the presence or absence of anomia evoked at various cortical sites is inversely related to the power of the electrocorticogram (ECoG) in this frequency band (Fried, Ojemann, and Fetz, 1981). These physiological changes are not seen when the same visual stimuli are used in a spatial matching paradigm. We thus have converging evidence for an association between naming and naming sites as determined by stimulation mapping. (See figure 30 and, for details, Fried et al., 1981, 1982; Oje-mann and Fried, 1982.)

The physiological changes keyed to naming (slow frontal negative shift, posterior desynchronization) are similar to the changes observed in experimental animals when the thalamocortical system is activated. A hypothesis to account for the human physiology, then, is that the frontal and pos-terior cortical areas are connected primarily via the thalamus, and not preferentially through corticocortical connections. Additionally, both anterior activity and posterior activity begin with the stimulus, indicating a parallel rather than a serial operation.

Electrophysiological data can be used on a trial-to-trial basis to determine whether activation of the cortex during naming, for example, is probabilistic (resulting in occasional functional failure) or is wired badly (resulting in error prone performance). A trial analysis for one patient in which the power in the 7–12-Hz band was plotted for fifteen trials at five posterior temporal and parietal sites, two of which were implicated by stimulation mapping as naming sites (Fried and Ojemann, unpublished data), showed that sites related to naming had least power in this band on 80 percent of trials with correct responses. But on 20 percent of these trials the least power, presumably representing maximal desynchronization, was not at sites that had shown changes in naming during stimulation mapping. This suggests that the physiological events at cortical sites related to a particular function have a probabilistic component, though the significance of this for performance remains to be determined.

When a subject produces overt vocal responses rather than silent naming, the slow negative shift is much more widespread and now most prominent in motor cortex. It is also evident in motor cortex of the nonlanguage dominant hemisphere.

Stimulation mapping can also be used to study organization of nondominant cortex. Labeling (identifying) the emotion expressed by a picture of a face is disrupted by stimulating in the right middle temporal gyrus in a fairly discrete location; subjects provided a name for an emotion, but the name given was different from the label chosen in control trials. Subjects were also able to identify faces correctly at these sites. Evidently, the deficit is not purely perceptual, but rather involves identification of facial emotions or more complex processing of spatial information (Fried et al., 1982).

Positron-emission-scan tomography (PET-scan) traces the metabolism of radioactive labeled 2-deoxyglucose. This substrate is metabolized like glucose, but does not break down in the brain, so that it pools there; 2-deoxyglucose also pools in the heart and bladder. The PET-scan procedure involves a 40–45-minute waiting period before isotope activity stabilizes; then six or more tomographic "slices" are counted, taking 10–15 minutes each. The computed slices reflect the metabolic activity of the brain over the entire period since the 2-deoxyglucose was administered. (The half-life of the radioactivity is 4–6 hours.) The slowness of the scanning procedure is not a problem with normal subjects, but makes it extremely difficult to use with dementing or hallucinating patients.

Gray matter and white matter can be clearly distinguished on the PET-scan printout, as can some of the subcortical structures; ventricle size can be gauged, but resolution still leaves much to be desired.

The effects of metabolic activity can be seen dramatically by comparing PET-scans of a normal subject taken (1) when the subject has spent the 45-minute period between injection of the drug and starting the scan procedure with eyes closed; (2) when the subject has spent the delay interval gazing at a gray ceiling illuminated with white light; and (3) when the subject has spent the interval outdoors watching busy campus pedestrian traffic. In the last instance, metabolic activity in the calcarine cortex is greatly enhanced.

Comparing PET-scans and x-ray CT-scans of aphasics, we find that stroke lesions usually seem larger on a PET-scan than on a CT-scan—for example, decreased cortical activity adjacent to a large posterior lesion in an aphasic was shown on a PET-scan, while the CT-scan showed only the deeper area of the lesion. Similarly, on the PET-scan and the CT-scan of a Wernicke's aphasic, only the PET-scan showed thalamic hypometabolism. Thalamic hypometabolism, as well as loss of function in Broca's area, has been observed also in a PET-scan taken on a patient with Broca's aphasia. On the other hand, a surgically caused lesion in a female patient who had had herpes encephalitis showed very similar CT- and PET-scans, without decreased thalamic activity, suggesting a difference between surgical and non-surgical lesions.

(The relation between lesions of the thalamus and aphasia is, incidentally, of some interest. Thalamic infarction may cause aphasia, but the aphasia is usually transient, even though the destructive lesion does not disappear. The role of the thalamus is probably not linguistic, but, rather, a general arousal of the cortex. If an aphasic had both thalamic and cortical hypometabolism but the thalamus returned to normal and the cortex did not, the aphasia would probably not remit.)

Two patients with thalamic hypometabolism were followed over time; one recovered from aphasia and one did not. The original PET-scan showed subcortical hypometabolism in both cases; the follow-up scan showed renewed metabolic activity in the patient who recovered, but not in the other. We can assume that the PET-scan reflects decreased activity when cells are present but not functioning; in contrast, x-ray CT-scans only show changes when cells are destroyed.

In conclusion, PET-scan is still a crude and difficult tool to use, but it has considerable potential. In general, the PET-scan is useful for detecting small discrete cerebral lesions, but is not good at dealing with large ones. New developments include a ten-"slice" series with an 8-millimeter resolution (ECAT); also, different radiopharmaceutical agents are being tested in a search for substances that will provide better responses. Researchers are devising appropriate tasks for subjects to carry out in the 45-minute period between administering the deoxyglucose and beginning the scanning— for example, comparing written and oral tasks.

PART VI

Concluding Comments

Electrical Stimulation Mapping

How are we to interpret the stimulation data? In particular, what is to be made of the association reported by Ojemann between disruptions in the ability to mimic sequences of orofacial movements and in the ability to identify stop consonants, evoked by stimulation at frontal, temporal, and parietal perisylvian sites? These findings seem to identify a cortical region that links speech perception to motor control in a fashion broadly consistent with a motor theory of speech perception (Liberman et al., 1967).

But the interpretation is not simple, since these results are in sharp disagreement with lesion data; deficits in phoneme and word identification are associated with damage to posterior temporal lobe (Wernicke's area), not to frontal (Broca's) or other perisylvian areas. Of course, many lesions have short-term effects quite different from their long-term effects; and, perhaps, if stimulation were sustained for a much longer time, the effects would be different. However, Darwin and his colleagues (Ettlinger, Teuber, and Milner, 1975, p. 132) have described a similar deficit in phoneme identification after resection of left face motor cortex—in patients, moreover, who were not aphasic—so that the transience of the stimulation is not likely to be relevant.

Perhaps the most plausible interpretation, at present, is that the task of phoneme identification calls for organization of a motor response in short-term memory by a process quite distinct from those of normal syllable or word perception and production. The fact that blockage may be induced by stimulation in orofacial areas not normally involved in speaking even suggests that the effect is essentially non-linguistic. Two responses, apparently identical in form, can be produced by different cortical systems if they have different functions. What we may have here, then, is a double dissociation between tasks and sites of lesion or stimulation; the normal linguistic task of lexical access is disrupted by posterior stimulation/lesion, while the metalinguistic mimicry (or production to command) of a meaningless stop consonant is blocked by stimulation/lesion in areas normally engaged for the organization of nonspeech orofacial movements.

In any event, the revival and refinement of the electrical stimulation technique promises a rich new source of data on localization. Like the grosser Wada sodium amytal test (Branch, Milner, and Rasmussen, 1964), stimulation mapping is validated by its success in predicting the effects of surgical resection. The next few years are likely to see a process of mutual accommodation and refinement in localization as the results from stimulation mapping and the new lesion scanning techniques (described by Benson) come in.

Relations between Lateralizations for Language and for Motor Control

The stimulation mapping results just discussed raise the general issue of the relation between movement control and language. The fact that both sequencing of movements (of hand and mouth) and language functions are disturbed by lesions of the left hemisphere does not necessarily mean that the two phenomena are causally related by some principle of economy, or efficiency, of processing. If this were so, we would expect individuals in whom language dominance and handedness are dissociated (for example, left-handers with left-hemisphere language) to display some manual or language deficit—which they do not. Moreover, as the patients of Darwin and his colleagues (Ettlinger, Teuber, and Milner, 1975) show, an individual may display disrupted orofacial motor sequencing, yet still be able to speak perfectly—and vice versa. In short, the familiar link between language and handedness is no more than a correlation; each function is the product of something else.

The "something else" may well be a general capacity of the left hemisphere for precise positioning and sequencing of movements, rooted in processes evolved for tool use, following the adoption of bipedalism (Lovejoy, 1981), some 3 1/2 million years ago. Speech and language seem to have exploited neural networks, already in place, to develop the rapid, informationally dense signaling system that an efficient communication system requires (compare Kimura, 1979; Studdert-Kennedy, 1981). To what extent speech and hand control still draw on shared neural organizations and mechanisms is, of course, an empirical issue (see, for example, Kinsbourne and Hicks, 1979; Lomas and Kimura, 1976; Lomas, 1980; Kelso, Tuller, and Harris, 1982). But it can hardly be an accident that the only articulatory system with a precision and agility to rival that of the vocal apparatus is in the hand—and that the hand, too, is an executor of language.

American Sign Language

The discovery of ASL, of its dual structure (formational and syntactic), its elaborate morphology, its complex embeddings of movements, and its underlying abstract forms—in fact, of the whole linguistic panoply that sets ASL on a par with spoken languages—encourages us to see the relations among movement control, handedness, and language function as a key to the perceptuomotor origins of language. We may even look to the instantiation of language in two different perceptuomotor modalities as the thin end of a wedge that may ultimately permit us to strip the modality from our descriptions and isolate language at the intersection of sign and speech. That intersection may well prove to be the common core of movement control from which a specialized syntactic capacity has evolved.

In the phonetic domain, specialized processes seem to be restricted to speech, and this is not surprising. The hands are capable of many more differentiable gestures than the vocal tract, and the eye can perhaps handle a finer and more varied range of information than the ear. We have perhaps had to evolve specialized mechanisms for extracting articulatory-phonetic information from speech sounds, but sign languages found mechanisms for reading signs already available in the visual system. If we had evolved for visual communication and were faced with the task of finding an auditory substitute for signs, we would probably find it impossible. The visual system readily adapts to a written alphabet, to finger-spelling or to the complex, interwoven structure of a sign language; but, as the history of attempts to substitute a sound alphabet for speech has shown (Studdert-Kennedy and Liberman, 1963), the auditory system is incapable of handling any sounds but those of speech at a rate fast enough for effective linguistic communication.

Granted the specialized phonetic and syntactic capacities vested for spoken languages in the left hemispheres of most individuals, we are led to wonder how sign language will prove to be localized. From Bellugi (see part IV) we already know that both fluent and nonfluent ASL aphasias result from left-hemisphere lesions, but we do not yet know the details of localization. Particularly interesting in this regard is Neville's (1977, 1980) evidence for evoked potentials in the *auditory* cortex of native signers in response to flashes of light. This points to extreme plasticity, as well as to neurological constraint on localization.

Evidently, within the limits of the left hemisphere, the human cortex is not rigidly wired. We depend on experience to establish the wiring. A normal infant, exposed to speech, develops the specialized perceptuomotor and linguistic systems for which the species is adapted; born deaf, and exposed to a sign language, the infant develops an alternative system no less readily. The concept of localization tempts us to think solely in terms of hardware, when, in fact, neural activity also forms around modes of operation shaped by the environment.

Does Structure Determine Function?

A recurrent controversy concerned the assumption implicit in studies of localization (whether by aphasic deficit or by stimulation mapping) that structure determines function. Suppose that we had ideal maps of brain activity, with resolution in space and time as sharp as we wanted, what could we then learn about how language is processed in the brain? The neural circuitry alone will not give us the program—any more than the circuitry of a computer reveals the range of programs that it can implement. We would have to work from known input/output relations, figuring out the functions necessary to yield those relations and comparing them with the circuits. Moreover, if computers are any guide, the relation of a particular deficit to a particular symptom can be far from obvious. If we are to learn about language processing from studies of aphasia, the form-function relations will have to be very much closer in humans than they are in computers. The gap between form and function is likely to be narrowest in the peripheral processes, widest in central or "higher" processes. It is the cognitively impenetrable functions, especially the more peripheral ones, that we are most likely to learn about from neuroanatomy and neurophysiology.

Finally, we should remember that there may be as much to be learned from computational models as from explicit neural speculations, even if these are based on sound physiological data. For example, if it is found that a particular cell fires whenever some event is perceived, we cannot conclude that this firing causes the percept. If perception depends on belief (as speech perception, for example, may depend on listening in a speech mode), and if the cell's firing only occurs after belief and stimulus are integrated, then the cell's activity is an index of perception, not a cause of it. In other words, correlations between neural activity and input/output events may tell us nothing about the processes that produce or follow from these events.

On the other hand, belief-contingent processes are not themselves beyond physiological investigation; Ojemann has observed changes in cortically evoked potentials from the language areas as a function of the instructions that a subject thinks he is following. The fact is that there are solid evolutionary grounds for expecting at least some degree of fit between form and function, and localization studies serve to place important constraints on models of how the neural circuitry works. Moreover, we would be unwise to reject a priori the possible contributions of neurology to an understanding of behavior—even of a behavior as complex as language. The history of the past fifty years offers many instances of advances in our understanding of behavior that have sprung from advances in our understanding of the behavior's physiological underpinnings.

For example, classical discussions of emotion often argued that emotions could not be understood on a physiological basis. One reason for this conclusion was that psychologists accepted natural language classifications of emotions and assumed homogeneity where there was none. However, a series of neurological findings, including the effects of destructive lesions, epilepsy in certain locations, and brain stimulation in human and other animals, demonstrated that certain specific emotions can be separated from the earlier gross categories and assigned specific locations in the brain.

Other examples come from vision. The classic paper of Lettvin et al. (1959) showed that visual analysis of form, at a very elementary level, might be carried out quite differently than had been thought; and the later studies of Hubel and Wiesel on cat cortex carried this revolution still further. Another instance is provided by color vision. Great advances were made by purely behavorial studies of input/output relations, but when it became possible to study the physiology of the cones and to measure the quantity of certain pigments in these cells, our understanding of color vision was revolutionized. In fact, the new knowledge of circuitry and biophotochemistry suggested new behavorial experiments that would not have been thought of before.

Similarly, in language, it would hardly have been possible to discover, by linguistic analysis, that commands for eye movements and commands for trunk movements might be dissociated in comprehension, as Geschwind reported earlier. This finding raises the possibility that certain modes of comprehension may have preceded others in the course of evolution and suggests new experiments to test this hypothesis.

In short, we do not have to define the behavior, do all the necessary behavorial studies, build a model of the input/output relations, and only then try to discover how the circuitry instantiates the models. Instead, we can look to an interaction between studies of behavior and studies of neural circuitry in which each style of research constrains and guides the other: Behavorial studies point to specific questions about the circuitry, and new understanding of the circuitry leads to new experiments on behavior.

Autonomy, Separability, and Specialization

The concept of autonomy is viewed quite differently by linguists, psychologists, and neurologists. For the linguist, autonomy of syntax or phonology, for example, simply refers to the fact that the formal apparatus of primitive terms and relations needed to describe the two subsystems are distinct and, indeed, incommensurable with respect both to one another and to other modes of cognition. Pylyshyn's notion of cognitive impenetrability is related to this linguistic view: Language—or, at least, certain subsystems within it—is incommensurate with, and therefore impervious to, the presumed propositional apparatus of general cognition (knowledge, beliefs, goals, intentions).

However, as soon as we consider how such formally distinct processes might be instantiated in the nervous system, the sharp distinctions begin to blur. Brain damage rarely, if ever, affects language alone. The recall of familiar sequences, the timing and sequencing of motion patterns, the ability to change set, the capacity to combine knowing and doing, all contribute to linguistic performance, and all may be damaged by brain lesions—or, for that matter, may be manipulated in psycholinguistic studies. Of course, this does not mean that separable subsystems within language do not exist; it means only that they are not readily isolated in practice. This serves to emphasize that all studies of brain activity in language function will be of dubious value until we can increase our knowledge of neural circuitry and place intelligent constraints on neural models of language.

Much of the difficulty arises from the fact that we are dealing with a system. Systems are conceptually recalcitrant because, by definition, they consist of parts that are both separable and connected. In other words, full autonomy of language, or its subsystems, is neurologically implausible. What we are more likely to find is a collection of specialized subsystems that more or less correspond to the linguist's descriptions, but are ultimately an integral part of the larger system. The most valuable contribution of neurology may not, in the end, be to validate linguistic description so much as to offer an approach to the deeper evolutionary question of how language relates to nonlanguage.

The task for the biologist is to derive the properties of language from the properties of its components. In other words, his task is to understand how language as a system emerged from some novel combination of more primitive, nonlinguistic mechanisms. For, as Jacob (1977, p. 1165) remarks of evolution: "It is always a matter of using the same elements, of adjusting them, of altering here or there, of arranging various combinations to produce new objects of increasing complexity. It is always a matter of tinkering."

Bibliography

Ahlgren, I., and Bergman, B., eds. (1980): Papers from: *First International Symposium on Sign Language Research*. (NATO Advanced Study Institute: Recent Developments in Language and Cognition. Copenhagen, Denmark.) Leksand, Sweden: Sveriges Dovas Riskforbund.

Andreewski, E., and Seron, X. (1975): Implicit processing of grammatical rules in a classical case of agrammatism. *Cortex* 11:379–390.

Arbib, M., and Caplan, D. (1979): Neurolinguistics must be computational. *Behav. Brain Sci.* 2:449–483.

Aronoff, M. (1976): *Word Formation in Generative Grammar*. (Linguistic Inquiry, Monograph 1.) Cambridge, MA: MIT Press.

Baker, C., and Cokely, D. (1980): *American Sign Language: A Teacher's Resource Text on Grammar and Culture*. Silver Spring, MD: National Association of the Deaf.

Baker, E., Blumstein, S., and Goodglass, H. (1981): Phonological vs. semantic factors in auditory comprehension. *Neuropsychologia* 19:1–15.

Bakker, D. J., and Moerland, R. (1981): Are there brain-tied sex differences in reading? In: *Sex Differences in Dyslexia*. Ansara, A., Geschwind, N., Galaburda, A., Albert, M., and Gartell, N., eds. Townson, MD: The Orton Dyslexia Society, pp. 109–117.

Barlow, G. B. (1977): Modal action patterns. In: *How Animals Communicate*. Sebeok, T. A., ed. Bloomington: Indiana University Press, pp. 98–134.

Barlow, G. B. (1981): Genetics and development of behavior, with special reference to patterned motor output. In: *Behavorial De-*

velopment. Immelmann, K., Barlow, G. B., Petrinovich, L., and Main, M., eds. Cambridge: Cambridge University Press, pp. 191–251.

Bates, E. (1976): *Language and Context.* New York: Academic Press.

Bates, E., Bretherton, I., Shore, C., and McNew, S. (1981): Names, gestures, and objects: Role of context in the emergence of symbols. In: *Children's Language,* vol. 4. Nelson, K. E., ed. New York: Halsted Press.

Bateson, P. P. G. (1976): Rules and reciprocity in behavioral development. In: *Growing Points in Ethology.* Bateson, P. P. G., and Hinde, R. A., eds. Cambridge: Cambridge University Press, pp. 401–421.

Bay, E. (1964): Classifications and concepts of aphasia. In: *Disorders of Language.* De Reuck, A. V. S., and O'Connor, M., eds. Boston: Little, Brown.

Bekoff, A. (1981): Embryonic development of the neural circuitry underlying motor coordination. In: *Studies in Developmental Neurobiology: Essays in Honor of Viktor Hamburger.* Cowan, W. M., ed. Oxford: Oxford University Press.

Bellugi, U. (1980a): The structuring of language: Clues from the similarities between signed and spoken language. In: *Signed and Spoken Language: Biological Constraints on Linguistic Form.* Bellugi, U., and Studdert-Kennedy, M., eds. (Dahlem Konferenzen) Weinheim: Verlag Chemie, pp. 115–140.

Bellugi, U. (1980b): How signs express complex meanings. In: *Sign Language and the Deaf Community, Essays in Honor of Wm. C. Stokoe.* Baker, C., and Battison, R., eds. Silver Spring, MD: National Association of the Deaf, pp. 53–74.

Bellugi, U., and Klima, E. S. (1980): Morphological processes in a language in a different mode. In: *The Elements: Linguistic Units and Levels.* Hands, W. F., Hofbauer, C., and Clyne, P. R., eds. Chicago: Chicago Linguistic Society, pp. 21–42.

Bellugi, U., and Klima, E. S. (1982): From gesture to sign: Deixis in a visual-gestural language. In: *Speech, Place and Action: Studies of Language in Context.* Jarvella, R. J., and Klein, W. eds., New York: John Wiley, pp. 297–313.

Bellugi, U., and Newkirk, D. (1980): Formal devices for creating new signs in American Sign Language. In: *Proceedings of the Na-*

tional Symposium on Sign Language Research and Teaching. Stokoe, W. C., ed. Silver Spring, MD: National Association of the Deaf, pp. 39–80.

Bellugi, U., and Studdert-Kennedy, M., eds. (1980): *Signed and Spoken Language: Biological Constraints on Linguistic Form.* (Dahlem Konferenzen) Weinheim: Verlag Chemie, pp. 115–140.

Bellugi, U., Klima, E. S., and Siple, P. (1975): Remembering in signs. *Cognition* 3:93–125.

Bellugi, U., Newkirk, D., Pedersen, C. C., and Fischer, S. (1979): The structured use of space and movement: Morphological processes. In: *The Signs of Language.* Klima, E. S., and Bellugi, U., eds. Cambridge, MA: Harvard University Press, pp. 272–398.

Bellugi, U., Poizner, H., and Zurif, E. (1982): Prospects for the study of aphasia in a visual-gestural language. In: *Neural Models of Language Processes.* Arbib, M. A., Caplan, D., and Marshall, J. C., eds. New York: Academic Press, pp. 271–292.

Benowitz, L. I., Bear, D. M., Rosenthal, R., Mesulam, M., Zaidel, E., and Sperry, R. W. (1982): Hemispheric specialization in nonverbal communication. *Science* (submitted).

Benson, D. F. (1977a): Neurologic correlates of aphasia and apraxia. In: *Recent Advances in Neurology,* vol. 2. Matthews, W. B., and Glaser, G. H., eds. London: Churchill-Livingstone.

Benson, D. F. (1977b): The third alexia. *Arch. Neurol.* 34:327–331.

Benson, D. F. (1979a): *Aphasia, Alexia and Agraphia.* New York: Churchill-Livingstone.

Benson, D. F. (1979b): Neurologic correlates of anomia. In: *Studies in Neurolinguistics,* vol. 4. Whitaker, H., and Whitaker, H., eds. New York: Academic Press, pp. 293–328.

Benson, D. F., and Geschwind, N. (1969): The alexias. In: *Handbook of Neurology,* vol. 4. Vinken, P. J., and Bruyn, G. W., eds. Amsterdam: North Holland, pp. 112–140.

Bentley, D. R. (1971): Genetic control of an insect neuronal network. *Science* 174:1139–1141.

Benton, A. L. (1980): The neuropsychology of facial recognition. *Am. Psychol.* 35:176–186.

Berlin, C. I., and McNeil, M. R. (1976): Dichotic listening. In: *Contemporary Issues in Experimental Phonetics.* Lass, N. J., ed. New York: Academic Press, pp. 327–387.

Berlucchi, G. (1974): Cerebral dominance and interhemispheric communication in normal man. In: *The Neurosciences: Third Study Program*. Schmitt, F. O., and Worden, F. G., eds. Cambridge, MA: MIT Press, pp. 65–69.

Berman, R. (1978): *Modern Hebrew Structure*. Tel Aviv: University Publishing Projects.

Berman, R. (1982): Verb-pattern alternation: The interface of morphology, syntax, and semantics in Hebrew child language. *J. Child Language* 9:169–192.

Berndt, R. S., and Caramazza, A. (1980): A redefinition of the syndrome of Broca's aphasia: Implications for a neuropsychological model of language. *Applied Psycholinguistics* 1:225–278.

Berndt, R. S., and Caramazza, A. (1981): Syntactic aspects of aphasia. In: *Acquired Aphasia*. Sarno, M. T., ed. New York: Academic Press, pp. 152–181.

Best, C. T., Morrongiello, B., and Robson, R. (1981): Perceptual equivalence of acoustic cues in speech and nonspeech perception. *Percept. Psychophys.* 29:191–211.

Bisiach, E. (1966): Perceptual factors in the pathogenesis of anomia. *Cortex* 2:90–95.

Blumstein, S., and Cooper, W. E. (1974): Hemispheric processing of intonation contours. *Cortex* 10:146–158.

Blumstein, S., Baker, E., and Goodglass, H. (1977): Phonological factors in auditory comprehension in aphasia. *Neuropsychologia* 15:19–30.

Blumstein, S., Cooper, W. E., Zurif, E., and Caramazza, A. (1977): The perception and production of voice-onset time in aphasia. *Neuropsychologia* 15:371–383.

Bogen, J. E., and Vogel, P. J. (1975): Neurologic status in the long term following complete cerebral commissurotomy. In: *Les Syndromes de Disconnexion Calleuse chez l'Homme*. Michel, F., and Schott, B., eds. Lyon: Hôpital Neurologique, pp. 227–251.

Boller, F., Kim, Y., and Mack, J. (1977): Auditory comprehension in aphasia. In: *Studies in Neurolinguistics*, vol. 3. Whitaker , H., and Whitaker, H., eds. New York: Academic Press.

Boyes-Braem, P. (1981): Features of the handshape in American Sign Language. PhD dissertation, University of California at Berkeley.

Bradley, D., Garrett, M., and Zurif, E. B. (1980): Syntactic deficits in Broca's aphasia. In: *Biological Studies of Mental Processes.* Caplan, D., ed. Cambridge, MA: MIT Press, pp. 269–286.

Bradshaw, J. L., and Nettleton, N. C. (1981): The nature of hemispheric specialization in man. *Brain Behav. Sci.* 4:51–91.

Branch, C., Milner, B., and Rasmussen, T. (1964): Intracarotid Amytal for the lateralization of cerebral speech dominance. *J. Neurosurg.* 21:399–405.

Bresnan, J. (1980): *The Passive in Lexical Theory.* Occasional Paper 7. Cambridge, MA: MIT Center for the Cognitive Sciences.

Cairns, H. S. (in press): Current issues in research in language comprehension. In: *Recent Advances in Language Sciences.* Naremore, R., ed. San Diego: College-Hill Press.

Caplan, D. (1980): Changing models of the neuropsychology of language. In: *Biological Studies of Mental Processes.* Caplan, D., ed. Cambridge, MA: MIT Press, pp. 234–238.

Caplan, D. (1981): On the cerebral localization of linguistic functions. *Brain Lang.* 14:120–137.

Caplan, D. (1982): Reconciling the categories: Representation in neurology and in linguistics. In: *Neural Models of Language Process.* Arbib, M. A., Caplan, D., and Marshall, J. C., eds. New York: Academic Press.

Caplan, D., and Chomsky, N. (1980): Linguistic perspectives on language development. In: *Biological Studies of Mental Processes.* Caplan, D., ed. Cambridge, MA: MIT Press, pp. 98–105.

Caplan, D., Matthei, E., and Gigley, H. (1981): Comprehension of gerundive constructions by Broca's aphasics. *Brain Lang.* 13:145–160.

Caramazza, A., and Berndt, R. B. (1978): Semantic and syntactic processes in aphasia: A review of the literature. *Psychol. Bull.* 85:898–918.

Caramazza, A., and Zurif, E. B. (1976): Dissociation of algorithmic and heuristic processes in language comprehension: Evidence from aphasia. *Brain Lang.* 3:572–582.

Caramazza, A., Berndt, R. S., and Brownell, H. (1982): The semantic deficit hypothesis: Perceptual parsing and object classification by aphasic patients. *Brain Lang.* 15:161–189.

Caramazza, A., Brownell, H., and Berndt, R. S. (1978): Naming and conceptual deficits in aphasia. Paper presented at: Academy of Aphasia, Chicago.

Caramazza, A., Berndt, R. S., Basili, A. G., and Koller, J. J. (1982): Syntactic processing deficits in aphasia. *Cortex* 17:333–347.

Caramazza, A., Gordon, J., Zurif, E. B., and DeLuca, D. (1976): Right-hemispheric damage and verbal problem-solving behavior. *Brain Lang.* 3:41–46.

Cavalli, M., DeRenzi, E., Fuglioni, P., and Vitale, A. (1981): Impairment of right brain-damaged patients on a linguistic cognitive task. *Cortex* 17:545–556.

Chiarello, C. (1981): Sign Language aphasia: A case study. Paper presented at: Academy of Aphasia, London, Ontario, October.

Chomsky, N. (1965): *Aspects of the Theory of Syntax.* Cambridge, MA: MIT Press.

Chomsky, N. (1970): Remarks on nominalization. In: *Readings in English.* Jacobs, R., and Rosenbaum, P., eds. Waltham, MA: Ginn.

Chomsky, N. (1980). *Rules and Representations.* New York: Columbia University Press.

Chomsky, N., and Halle, M. (1968): *The Sound Pattern of English.* New York: Harper & Row.

Coltheart, M. (1980): Deep dyslexia: A right hemisphere hypothesis. In: *Deep Dyslexia.* Coltheart, M., Patterson, K., and Marshall, J. C., eds. London: Routledge and Kegan Paul.

Coltheart, M., Patterson, K., and Marshall, J. C., eds. (1980): *Deep Dyslexia.* London: Routledge and Kegan Paul.

Cooper, W. E. (1980): Intonation in agrammatism. Paper presented at: Academy of Aphasia, Bass River, MA.

Cooper, W. E., and Zurif, E. B. (1981): Comprehension and production in language pathology. In: *Language Production*, vol. 11. Butterworth, B., ed. London: Academic Press.

Critchley, M. (1962): Speech and speech loss in relation to duality of the brain. In: *Interhemispheric Relations and Cerebral Dominance.* Mountcastle, V. B., ed. Baltimore: Johns Hopkins University Press, pp. 208–213.

Cummings, J. L., Benson, D. F., Walsh, M. J., and Levine, H. L. (1979): Left-to-right transfer of language dominance: A case study. *Neurology* 29:1547–1549.

Czopf, J. (1972): Uber die Rolle der nicht dominant Hemisphare in der Restitution der Sprache der Aphasischen. *Archiv für Psychiatrie und Nervenkrankheiten* 216:162–171.

Dawkins, R. (1976): Hierarchical organisation: A candidate principle for ethology. In: *Growing Points in Ethology.* Bateson, P. P. G., and Hinde, R. A., eds. Cambridge: Cambridge University Press, pp. 7–54.

Day, J. (1977): Right-hemispheric language processing in normal right-handers. *J. Exp. Psychol.* (Human Perception and Performance) 3:518–528.

Day, J. (1979): Visual half-field word recognition as a function of syntactic class and imageability. *Neuropsychologia* 17:515–519.

Dennis, M. (1980a): Capacity and strategy for syntactic comprehension after left or right hemidecortication. *Brain Lang.* 10:287–317.

Dennis, M. (1980b): Language acquisition in a single hemisphere: Semantic organization. In: *Biological Studies of Mental Processes.* Caplan, D., ed. Cambridge, MA: MIT Press, pp. 159–185.

Dennis, M. (1980c): Strokes in childhood. I. Communicative intent, expression, and comprehension after left hemisphere arteriopathy in a right-handed nine-year-old. In: *Language Development and Aphasia in Children.* Rieber, R., ed. New York: Academic Press, pp. 45–67.

Dennis, M., and Kohn, B. (1975): Comprehension of syntax in infantile hemiplegics after cerebral hemidecortication: Left hemisphere superiority. *Brain Lang.* 2: 472–482.

Dennis, M., and Lovett, M. (1982): The acquisition of story schemas in the two sides of the brain. Manuscript.

Dennis, M., and Whitaker, H. A. (1976): Language acquisition following hemidecortication: Linguistic superiority of the left over the right hemisphere. *Brain Lang.* 3:404–433.

Dennis, M., Lovett, M., and Wiegel-Crump, C. A. (1981): Written language acquisition after left or right hemidecortication in infancy. *Brain Lang.* 12:54–91.

Dennis, M., Newman, J., and Lovett, M. (1982): Referential cohesion in the story-telling of the two hemispheres. Manuscript.

De Renzi, E., and Spinnler, H. (1967): Impaired performance on color tasks in patients with hemispheric damage. *Cortex* 3:194–217.

Dodd, B. (1979): Lip reading in infants: Attention to speech presented in- and out-of-synchrony. *Cognitive Psychology* 11:478–484.

Efron, R. (1963): Temporal perception, aphasis and déjà vu. *Brain* 86:403–424.

Ettlinger, G., Teuber, H.-L., and Milner, B. (1975): The Seventeenth International Symposium of Neuropsychology. *Neuropsychologia* 13:125–134.

Fentress, J. C. (1972): Development and patterning of movement sequences in inbred mice. In: *The Biology of Behavior.* Kiger, J., ed. Corvallis, Oregon: Oregon State University Press, pp. 83–132.

Fentress, J. C. (1973): Development of grooming in mice with amputated forelimbs. *Science* 179:704–705.

Fentress, J. C. (1976): Dynamic boundaries of patterned behaviour: Interaction and self-organization. In: *Growing Points in Ethology.* Bateson, P. P. G., and Hinde, R. A., eds. Cambridge: Cambridge University Press, pp. 135–169.

Fentress, J. C. (1977): The tonic hypothesis and the patterning of behavior. *Annals N.Y. Acad. Sci.* 290:370–395.

Fentress, J. C. (1978): Mus musicus: The developmental orchestration of selected movement patterns in mice. In: *The Development of Behavior: Comparative and Evolutionary Aspects.* Burghardt, G. M., and Bekoff, M., eds. New York: Garland Press, pp. 321–342.

Fentress, J. C. (1980): How can behavior be studied from a neuroethological perspective? In: *Information Processing in the Nervous System.* Pinsker, H. M., and Willis, W. D., Jr., eds. New York: Raven Press, pp. 263–283.

Fentress, J. C. (1981a): Order in ontogeny: Relational dynamics. In: *Behavorial Development.* Immelmann, K., Barlow, G., Main, M., and Petrinovich, L., eds. Cambridge: Cambridge University Press, pp. 338–371.

Fentress, J. C. (1981b): Sensorimotor development. In: *The Development of Perception: Psychobiological Perspectives,* vol. 1. Aslin, R. N., Alberts, J. R., and Petersen, M. R., eds. New York: Academic Press, pp. 293–318.

Fentress, J. C. (1982): Ethological models of hierarchy and patterning of species-specific behavior. In: *Handbook of Neurobiology: Motivation*. Satinoff, E., and Teitelbaum, P., eds. New York: Plenum Press.

Fentress, J. C., and Stilwell, F. P. (1973): Grammar of a movement sequence in inbred mice. *Nature* 244:52–53.

Field, T. M., Woodson, R., Greenberg, R., and Cohen, D. (1982): Discrimination and imitation of facial expressions by neonates. *Science* 218:179–181.

Fillmore, C. (1968): The case for case. In: *Universals of Linguistic Structure*. Bach, E., and Harms, R. H., eds. New York: Holt, Rinehart and Winston.

Fitch, H. L., Halwes, T., Erickson, D. M., and Liberman, A. M. (1980): Perceptual equivalence of two acoustic cues for stop-consonant manner. *Percept. Psychophys.* 27:343–350.

Fodor, J. A., Bever, T. G., and Garrett, M. F. (1974): *The Psychology of Language*. New York: McGraw-Hill.

Fodor, J. A., Garrett, M. F., Walker, E. C. T., and Parkes, C. H. (1980): Against definitions. *Cognition* 8:263–367.

Fokjaer-Jensen, B., ed. (1980): *Recent Developments in Language and Cognition* (special edition of *Logos*). Copenhagen: University of Denmark.

Forster, K. (1979): Levels of processing and the structure of the language processor. In: *Sentence Processing: Psycholinguistic Studies Presented to Merrill Garrett*. Cooper, W. E., and Walker, E. C. T., eds. Hillsdale, NJ: Lawrence Erlbaum, pp. 27–85.

Foss, D. J. (1969): Decision processes during sentence comprehension: Effects of lexical item difficulty and position upon decision times. *J. Verb. Learn. Verb. Behav.* 8:457–462.

Foss, D. J. (1970): Some effects of ambiguity upon sentence comprehension. *J. Verb. Learn. Verb. Behav.* 9:699–706.

Franz, S. I. (1933): The inadequacy of the concept of unilateral cerebral dominance in learning. *J. Exp. Psychol.* 16:873–875.

Franz, S. I., and Davis, E. F. (1933): Simultaneous reading with both cerebral hemispheres. In: *Studies in Cerebral Function, IV*. (Publications of the University of California at Los Angeles in Education, Philosophy and Psychology, vol. 1, pp. 96–106.)

Franz, S. I., and Kilduff, S. (1933): Cerebral dominance as shown by segmental visual learning. In: *Studies in Cerebral Function, II.* (Publications of the University of California at Los Angeles in Education, Philosophy and Psychology, vol. 1, pp. 79–90.)

Fried, I., Ojemann, G. A., and Fetz, E. E. (1981): Language-related potentials specific to human language cortex. *Science* 212:353–355.

Fried, I., Mateer, C., Ojemann. G., Wohns, R., and Fedio, P. (1982): Organization of visuospatial functions in human cortex: Evidence from electrical stimulation. *Brain* 105:349–371.

Friederici, A. (1982): Syntactic and semantic processes in aphasic deficits: The availability of prepositions. *Brain Lang.* 15:249–258.

Friedman, A., and Poulson, M. C. (1981): The hemispheres as independent resource-systems: Limited-capacity processing and cerebral specialization. *J. Exp. Psychol. (Human Perception and Performance)* 7:1031–1058.

Frishberg, N. (1975): Arbitrariness and iconicity: Historical change in American Sign Language. *Language* 51:696–719.

Frost, N. (1972): Encoding and retrieval in visual memory tasks. *J. Exp. Psychol.* 95:317–326.

Gainotti, G., Calagirone, C., Micei, G., and Masullo, C. (1981): Selective semantic-lexical impairment of language comprehension in right-brain-damaged patients. *Brain Lang.* 13:201–211.

Galaburda, A. M., and Kemper, T. L. (1979): Cytoarchitectonic abnormalities in developmental dyslexia: A case study. *Ann. Neurol.* 6:94.

Galaburda, A. M., Sanides, F., and Geschwind, N. (1978): Human brain: Cytoarchitectonic left-right asymmetries in the temporal speech region. *Arch. Neurol.* 35:812–817.

Galaburda, A. M., LeMay, M., Kemper, T. L., and Geschwind, N. (1978): Right-left asymmetries in the brain. Structural differences between the hemispheres may underlie cerebral dominance. *Science* 199:852–856.

Gardner, H., and Denes, G. (1973): Connotative judgments by aphasic patients on a pictorial adoptation of the semantic differential. *Cortex* 9:183–196.

Gardner, H., Ling, P. K., Flamm, L., and Silverman, J. (1975): Comprehension and appreciation of humorous material following brain damage. *Brain* 98:399–412.

Gardner, H., Silverman, J., Wapner, W., and Zurif, E. (1978): The appreciation of antonymic contrast in aphasia. *Brain Lang.* 6:301–317.

Garrett, M. (1981): Objects of psycholinguistic enquiry. *Cognition* 10:97–101.

Garrett, M. (1982): Production of speech: Observations from normal and pathological language use. In: *Normality and Pathology in Cognitive Functions.* Ellis, A. W., ed. London: Academic Press.

Gazzaniga, M. S. (1970): *The Bisected Brain.* New York: Appleton-Century-Crofts.

Gazzaniga, M. S., and LeDoux, J. (1978): *The Integrated Mind.* New York: Plenum Press.

Geffen, G., Traub, E., and Stierman, I. (1978): Language laterality assessed by unilateral ECT and dichotic monitoring. *Journal of Neurology, Neurosurgery, and Psychiatry* 41:354–360.

Gentner, D. (1976): Evidence for the psychological reality of semantic components: The verbs of possession. In: *Explorations in Cognition.* Norman, D. A., and Rumelhart, D. E., eds. San Francisco: Freeman.

Geschwind, N. (1964): The development of the brain and the evolution of language. Monograph Series on Language and Linguistics 17. Washington, DC: Georgetown University Press, pp. 155–169.

Geschwind, N. (1965): Disconnexion syndromes in animals and man. *Brain* 88:237–294.

Geschwind, N. (1970): Organization of language and the brain. *Science* 170:940–944.

Geschwind, N. (1974): Late changes in the nervous system: An overview. In: *Plasticity and Recovery of Function in the Central Nervous System.* Stein, D., and Rosen, J., eds. New York: Academic Press, pp. 467–508.

Geschwind, N. (1975): The apraxias: Neural mechanisms of disorders of learned movement. *Am. Sci.* 63:188–195.

Geschwind, N., and Kaplan, E. (1962): A human cerebral deconnection syndrome. *Neurobiology* 12:675–685.

Geschwind, N., and Levitsky, W. (1968): Human brain: Left-right asymmetries in temporal speech region. *Science* 161:186–187.

Golani, I. (1976): Homeostatic motor processes in mammalian interactions: A choreography of display. In: *Perspectives in Ethology*, vol. 2. Bateson, P. P. G., and Klopfer, P. H., eds. New York: Plenum Press, pp. 69–134.

Golani, I. (1981): The search for invariants in motor behavior. In: *Behavorial Development*. Immelmann, K., Barlow, G., Main, M., and Petrinovich, L., eds. Cambridge: Cambridge University Press, pp. 372–390.

Goldman, P. S., and Galkin, T. W. (1978): Prenatal removal of frontal association cortex in the fetal rhesus monkey: Anatomical and functional consequences in postnatal life. *Brain Res.* 152:451–485.

Goldstein, K. (1948): *Language and Language Disturbances.* New York: Grune and Stratton.

Goodglass, H. (1968): Studies in the grammar of aphasics. In: *Developments in Applied Psychological Research.* Rosenburg, S., and Koplin, J., eds. New York: Macmillan.

Goodglass, H. (1980a): Disorders of naming following brain injury. Observation of the effects of brain injury adds another dimension to our understanding of the relations between neurological and psychological factors in the naming process. *Am. Sci.* 68:647–655.

Goodglass, H. (1980b): Word-finding in aphasia. Paper presented at: Academy of Aphasia, Bass River, MA.

Goodglass, H., and Baker, E. (1976): Semantic field, naming, and auditory comprehension in aphasia. *Brain Lang.* 3:359–374.

Goodglass, H., and Geschwind, N. (1976): Language disturbance (aphasia). In: *Handbook of Perception*, vol. 7. Carterette, E. C., and Friedman, M. P., eds. New York: Academic Press.

Goodglass, H., and Hunt, J. (1958): Grammatical complexity and aphasic speech. *Word* 14:197–207. (Reprinted in: *Selected Papers in Neurolinguistics.* Peuser, G., ed. München: Wilhelm Fink Verlag, 1978.)

Goodglass, H., and Hunter, M. (1970): A linguistic comparison of speech and writing in two types of aphasia. *Communication Disorders* 3:28–35.

Goodglass, H., and Kaplan, E. (1963): Disturbance of gesture and pantomime in aphasia. *Brain* 86:703–720.

Goodglass, H., and Kaplan, E. (1972): *The Assessment of Aphasia and Related Disorders*. Philadelphia: Lea and Febiger.

Goodglass, H., and Stuss, D. T. (1979): Naming to picture versus description in three aphasic subgroups. *Cortex* 15:199–211.

Goodglass, H., Kaplan, E., Weintraub, S., and Ackerman, N. (1976): The tip-of-the-tongue phenomenon in aphasia. *Cortex* 12:145–153.

Goodglass, H., Blumstein, S. E., Gleason, J. B., Hyde, M. R., Green, E., and Statlender, S. (1979): The effect of syntactic encoding on sentence comprehension in aphasia. *Brain Lang.* 7:201–209.

Gowers, W. R. (1887): *Lectures on the Diagnosis of Diseases of the Brain*. London: Churchill.

Haas, M. R. (1977): Tonal accent in Creek. In: *Studies in Stress and Accent*. Southern California Occasional Papers in Linguistics No. 4. USC Linguistics Department. Los Angeles: University of California Press.

Haggard, M. P., and Parkinson, A. M. (1971): Stimulus task factors as determinants of ear advantages. *Quarterly J. Exp. Psychol.* 23:168–177.

Halle, M. (1973): Prolegomena to a theory of word formation. *Linguistic Inquiry* 4:3–16.

Halle, M., and Vergnaud, J. R. (1980): Three-dimensional phonology. Manuscript. MIT.

Head, H. (1926): *Aphasia and Kindred Disorders of Speech*. Cambridge: Cambridge University Press.

Hebb, D. O. (1953): Heredity and environment in mammalian behaviour. *Br. J. Animal Behaviour* 1:43–47.

Hecaen, H., and Albert, M. L. (1978): *Human Neuropsychology*. New York: Wiley-Interscience.

Heeschen, C. (1980): Strategy of decoding actor-object-relations by aphasic patients. *Cortex* 16:5–19.

Heilman, K. M., and Scholes, R. J. (1976): The nature of comprehension errors in Broca's, conduction, and Wernicke's aphasics. *Cortex* 12:258–265.

Heilman, K. M., Scholes, R., and Watson, R. (1975): Auditory affective agnosia. *J. Neurol. Neurosurg. Psychiatr.* 38:69–72.

Hellige, J. B., and Cox, P. J. (1976): Effects of concurrent verbal memory on recognition of stimuli from the left and right visual fields. *J. Exp. Psychol. (Human Perception and Performance)* 2:210–221.

Hellige, J. B., Cox, P. J., and Litvak, L. (1979): Information processing in cerebral hemispheric activation and capacity. *J. Exp. Psychol.* 108:251–279.

Hoffmeister, R. (1975): The development of demonstrative pronouns, locatives, and personal pronouns in the acquisition of American Sign Language by deaf children of deaf parents. PhD dissertation. University of Minnesota.

Hoffmeister, R. (1978): An analysis of possessive constructions in the ASL of a young deaf child of deaf parents. In: *Sign Language Research.* Wilbur, R., ed. (Special issue of *Communication and Cognition.*)

Hoffmeister, R., and Wilbur, R. (1980): Developmental: The acquisition of sign language. In: *Recent Perspectives on American Sign Language.* Lane, H., and Grosjean, F., eds. Hillsdale, NJ: Lawrence Erlbaum.

Hubel, D. H., and Wiesel, T. N. (1962): Receptive fields, binocular interaction and functional architecture in the cat's visual cortex. *J. Physiol.* 60:106–154.

Huxley, J. S. (1914): The courtship habits of the great crested grebe (*Podiceps cristatus*), with an addition on the theory of sexual selection. *Proc. Zool. Soc.* (London): 491–562.

Jaccarino, G. (1975): Dual encoding in memory. Evidence from temporal-lobe lesions in man. MA thesis. McGill University.

Jackendoff, R. (1978): Toward an explanatory semantic representation. *Linguistic Inquiry* 7:89–150.

Jacob, F. (1977): Evolution as tinkering. *Science* 196:1161–1166.

Jones, M. K. (1976): Imagery as a mnemonic aid after left temporal lobectomy; contrast between specific and generalized memory disorders. *Neuropsychologia* 12:21–30.

Jones-Gotman, M. (1979): Incidental learning of image mediated or pronounced words after right temporal lobectomy. *Cortex* 15:187–198.

Jones-Gotman, M. and Milner, B. (1974): Right temporal-lobe contribution to language mediated verbal learning. *Neuropsychologia* 16:61–71.

Kantor, R. (1982): Communicative interaction in American Sign Language between deaf mothers and their deaf children: A psycholinguistic analysis. PhD dissertation. Boston University.

Katz, J. J., and Fodor, J. A. (1964): The structure of a semantic theory. In: *The Structure of Language*. Katz, J., and Fodor, J., eds. Englewood Cliffs, NJ: Prentice-Hall.

Kean, M. L. (1981): Grammatical representations and the description of linguistic processing. In: *Biological Studies of Mental Processes*. Caplan, D., ed. Cambridge, MA: MIT Press.

Kelso, S., Tuller, B., and Harris, K. S. (1982): A "dynamic pattern" perspective on the control and coordination of movement. In: *The Production of Speech*. MacNeilage, P., ed. New York: Springer.

Kent, R. D. (1981): Sensorimotor aspects of speech development. In: *The Development of Perception: Psychobiological Perspectives*, vol. 1. Aslin, R. N., Alberts, J. R., and Petersen, M. R., eds. New York: Academic Press, pp. 161–189.

Kimball, J. (1973): Seven principles of surface structure parsing in natural language. *Cognition* 2:15–47.

Kimball, J. (1975): Predictive analysis and over-the-top parsing. In: *Syntax and Semantics*, vol. 4. Kimball, J., ed. New York: Academic Press.

Kimura, D. (1976): The neural basis of language *qua* gesture. In: *Studies in Neurolinguistics*, vol. 2. Whitaker, H., and Whitaker, H. A., eds. New York: Academic Press, pp. 145–156.

Kimura, D. (1979): Neuromotor mechanisms in the evolution of human communication. In: *Neurobiology of Social Communication in Primates*. Steklis, H. D., and Raleigh, M. J., eds. New York: Academic Press, pp. 197–219.

Kimura, D. (1982): Neural mechanisms in manual signing. *Sign Language Studies* 33:291–312.

Kimura, D., and Durnford, M. (1974): Normal studies on the function of the right hemisphere in vision. In: *Hemisphere Function in the Human Brain*. Diamond, S. J., and Beaumont, J. G., eds. London: Elek Scientific Books, pp. 25–47.

Kinsbourne, M. (1971): The minor cerebral hemisphere as a source of aphasic speech. *Arch. Neurol.* 25:302–306.

Kinsbourne, M., and Hicks, R. E. (1979): Mapping cerebral functional space: Competition and collaboration in human performance. In: *Asymmetrical Function of the Brain*. Kinsbourne, M., ed. Cambridge: Cambridge University Press, pp. 267–273.

Klatt, D. H., and Stefanski, R. A. (1974): How does a mynah bird imitate human speech? *J. Acoust. Soc. Amer.* 55:82–89.

Klein, B. (1978): Inferring functional localization from neurological evidence. In: *Explorations in the Biology of Language*. Walker, E., ed. Montgomery, VT: Bradford Books.

Klima, E. S., and Bellugi, U. (1976): Poetry and song in a language without sound. *Cognition* 4:45–97.

Klima, E. S., and Bellugi, U. (1979): *The Signs of Language*. Cambridge, MA: Harvard University Press.

Kohn, B. (1980): Right-hemisphere speech representation and comprehension of syntax after left cerebral injury. *Brain Lang.* 9:350–361.

Kohn, S., Schonle, P. W., and Hawkins, W. (1982): Identification of pictured homonyms. Latent phonological knowledge in Broca's aphasia. Manuscript.

Kolk, H. (1978): Judgment of sentence structure in Broca's aphasia. *Neuropsychologia* 16:617–625.

Kolk, H. (1981): Nonsyntactic sources of agrammatism. Paper presented at: Academy of Aphasia, London, Ontario.

Krantz, G. S. (1980): Sapientization and speech. *Current Anthropology* 21:773–792.

Kuhl, P. K., and Meltzoff, A. N. (1982): The bimodal perception of speech in infancy. *Science* 218:1138–1144.

Kuhl, P. K., and Miller, J. D. (1978): Speech perception by the chinchilla: Identification functions for synthetic VOT stimuli. *J. Acoust. Soc. Amer.* 63:905–917.

Ladefoged, P. (1980): What are linguistic sounds made of? *Language* 56: 485–502.

Lane, H., and Grosjean, F. (1980): *Recent Perspectives on American Sign Language*. Hillsdale, NJ: Lawrence Erlbaum.

Lashley, K. S. (1951): The problem of serial order in behavior. In: *Cerebral Mechanisms in Behavior*. Jeffress, L. A., ed. New York: John Wiley, pp. 112–136.

Launer, P. (1982): "A plane" is not "To fly": Acquiring the distinction between related nouns and verbs in American Sign Language. Unpublished PhD dissertation. City University of New York.

Lenneberg, E. H. (1967): *Biological Foundations of Language*. New York: John Wiley.

Lenneberg, E. H. (1974): Language and brain: Developmental aspects. *Neurosci. Res. Prog. Bull.* 12:511–656.

Lesser, R. (1974): Verbal comprehension in aphasia: An English version of three Italian tests. *Cortex* 10:247–263.

Lettvin, J. Y., Maturana, H. R., McCulloch, W. S., and Pitts, W. H. (1959): What the frog's eye tells the frog's brain. *Proc. I.R.E.* 47:1940–1951.

Lévi-Strauss, J. (1966): *The Savage Mind*. Chicago: University of Chicago Press.

Levy, J. (1974): Psychobiological implications of bilateral symmetry. In: *Hemisphere Function in the Human Brain*. Dimond, S. J., and Beaumont, J. G., eds. New York: Halsted Press, pp. 121–183.

Levy, J. (1982): Mental processes in the nonverbal hemisphere. In: *Animal Mind—Human Mind*. Griffin, D. R., ed. Heidelberg: Springer-Verlag.

Levy, J., and Trevarthen, C. (1977): Perceptual, semantic, and phonetic aspects of elementary language processes in split brain patients. *Brain* 100: 105–118.

Liberman, A. M. (1970): The grammars of speech and language. *Cognitive Psychology* 1:301–323.

Liberman, A. M. (1980): An ethological approach to language through the study of speech perception. In: *Human Ethology*. Cranach, M. von, Foppa, K., Lepenies, W., and Ploog, D., eds. Cambridge: Cambridge University Press, pp. 682–704.

Liberman, A. M., and Studdert-Kennedy, M. (1978): Phonetic perception. In: *Handbook of Sensory Physiology*, vol. VIII: *Perception*. Held, R., Leibowitz, H., and Teuber, H.-L., eds. Heidelberg: Springer-Verlag, pp. 144–178.

Liberman, A. M., Isenberg, D., and Rakerd, B. (1981): Duplex perception of cues for stop consonants: Evidence for a phonetic mode. *Percept. & Psychophys.* 30:133–141.

Liberman. A. M., Cooper, F., Shankweiler, D., and Studdert-Kennedy, M. (1967): Perception of the speech code. *Psychol. Rev.* 74:431–461.

Liddell, S. K. (1980): *American Sign Language Syntax*. The Hague: Mouton.

Lieber, R. (1980): The organization of the lexicon. PhD dissertation. Department of Linguistics and Philosophy, MIT.

Lieberman, P. (1980): On the development of vowel production in young children. In: *Child Phonology*, vol. 1: *Production*. Yeni-Komshian, G. H., Kavanagh, J. F., and Ferguson, C. A., eds. New York: Academic Press, pp. 113–142.

Lindblom, B., and Sundberg, J. (1971): Neurophysiological representation of speech sounds. Paper presented at: XVth World Congress of Logopedics and Phoniatrics, Buenos Aires, Argentina, August 14–19.

Lindblom, B., Lubker, J., and Gay, T. (1979): Formant frequencies of some fixed-mandible vowels and a model of speech motor programming by predictive simulation. *J. Phonetics* 7:147–161.

Lineberger, M., Schwartz, M., and Saffran, E. (1981): Grammaticality judgments of agrammatic aphasia. Paper presented at: BABBLE , Niagara Falls, Ontario

Loew, R. C. (1982): Roles and reference. In: *Proceedings of the Third National Symposium on Sign Language Research and Teaching*. Caccamise, F., Garretson, M., and Bellugi, U., eds. Silver Spring, MD: National Association of the Deaf.

Lomas, J. (1980): Competition within the left hemisphere between speaking and unimanual tasks performed without visual guidance. *Neuropsychologia* 18:141–150.

Lomas, J., and Kimura, D. (1976): Intrahemispheric interaction between speaking and manual action. *Neuropsychologia* 14:23–33.

Lovejoy, C. O. (1981): The origin of man. *Science* 211:341–350.

Luria, A. R. (1947): *Traumatic Aphasia: Its Syndromes, Psychology and Treatment*. Moscow: Izd. Akad. Meditsin Nauk SSSR. (Reprinted in The Hague: Mouton, 1970; translated from the Russian by Douglas Bowden.)

Luria, A. R. (1976): *Basic Problems in Neurolinguistics*. The Hague: Mouton.

McCarthy, J. (1979): Formal problems in semitic phonology and morphology. PhD. dissertation. MIT.

MacDonald, J., and McGurk, H. (1978): Visual influences on speech perception processes. *Percept. & Psychophys.* 24:253–257.

McGurk, H., and MacDonald, J. (1976): Hearing lips and seeing voices. *Nature* 264:746.

McIntire, M. (1977): The acquisition of American Sign Language. *Sign Language Studies* 16:247–266.

MacKain, K., Studdert-Kennedy, M., Spikeer, S., and Stern, D. (in press): Intermodal speech perception in infants is a left hemisphere function. *Science.*

McKeeves, W. F., and Suberi, M. (1974): Parallel but temporary displaced visual half-field metacontrast functions. *Quart. J. Exp. Psychol.* 26:258–265.

MacNeilage, P. F. (1970): Motor control of serial ordering of speech. *Psychol. Rev.* 77:182–196.

Madden, D. J., and Nebes, R. D. (1980): Visual perception and memory. In: *The Brain and Psychology*. Wittrock, M. C., ed. New York: Academic Press.

Madden, D. J., Nebes, R. B., and Berg, W. D. (1981): Signal detection analysis of hemispheric differences in visual recognition memory. *Cortex* 17:491–502.

Marin, O., Saffran, E. M., and Schwartz, M. F. (1976): Dissociations of language in aphasia: Implications for normal function. *Annals N.Y. Acad. Sci.* 280:868–884.

Marler, P., and Peters, S. (1977): Selective vocal learning in a sparrow. *Science* 198:519–521.

Marshall, J. C., and Newcombe, F. (1973): Patterns of paralexia: A psycholinguistic approach. *J. Psycholinguistics* 2:175–199.

Mateer, C., and Kimura, D. (1977): Impairment of non-verbal oral movements in aphasia. *Brain Lang.* 4:262–276.

Mateer, C., Polen, S., Ojemann, G., and Wyler, A. (1982): Cortical localization of finger spelling and oral language: A case study. *Brain Lang.* 17:46–57.

Maxwell, M. (1980): Language acquisition in a deaf child: The interaction of sign variations, speech, and print variations. PhD. dissertation. University of Arizona.

Meadows, J. C. (1974): The anatomical basis of prosopagnosia. *J. Neurol. Neurosurg. Psychiatr.* 37:489–501.

Meier, R. (1981): Icons and morphemes: Models of the acquisition of verb agreement. *Papers and Reports on Child Language Development* 20:92–99.

Meier, R. (1982): Icons, analogues, and morphemes: The acquisition of verb agreement in American Sign Language. PhD dissertation. University of California at San Diego.

Meltzoff, A. N., and Moore, M. K. (1977): Imitation of facial and manual gestures by human neonates. *Science* 198:175–178.

Miceli, G., Menn, L., Mazzucchi, A., and Goodglass, H. (1981): Two case studies. Paper presented at: BABBLE, Niagara Falls, Ontario.

Miller, G. A. (1951): *Language and Communication.* New York: McGraw-Hill.

Miller, G. A. (1978): Lexical meaning. In: *Speech and Language in the Laboratory, School and Clinic.* Kavanaugh, J. F., and Strange, W., eds. Cambridge, MA: MIT Press.

Miller, G. A., and Johnson-Laird, P. (1976): *Language and Perception.* Cambridge, MA: Harvard University Press. ·

Milner, B. (1978): Clues to cerebral organization. In: *Cerebral Correlates of Conscious Experience.* Buser, P. A., and Rougeul-Buser, A., eds. Amsterdam: North Holland.

Mishkin, M., and Forgays, D. G. (1952): Word recognition as a function of retinal locus. *J. Exp. Psychol.* 43:43–48.

Mohr, J. (1976): Broca's area and Broca's aphasia. *Studies in Neurolinguistics* 1:201–236.

Morais, J. (1982): The two sides of cognition. In: *Perspectives in Mental Representation.* Mehler, J., Walker, E. C. T., and Garrett, M., eds. Hillsdale, NJ: Lawrence Erlbaum, pp. 277–309.

Moscovitch, M. (1973): Language and the cerebral hemispheres: Reaction-time studies and their implications for models of cerebral dominance. In: *Communication and Affect: Language and Thought.*

Pliner, P., Alloway, T., and Krames, L., eds. New York: Academic Press, pp. 89–126.

Moscovitch, M. (1976): On the representation of language in the right hemisphere of right-handed people. *Brain Lang.* 3:47–71.

Moscovitch, M. (1979): Information processing and the cerebral hemispheres. In: *Handbook of Behavioral Neurobiology*, vol. 2. Gazzaniga, M. S., ed. New York: Plenum Press, pp. 379–446.

Moscovitch, M. (1981): Right hemisphere language. *Topics in Language Disorders* 1:41–61.

Moscovitch, M., and Catlin, J. (1970): Interhemispheric transmission of information: Measurement in normal man. *Psychonom. Sci.* 18:211–213.

Moscovitch, M., and Klein, D. (1980): Material-specific perceptual interference for visual words and faces: Implications for models of capacity limitations, attention, and laterality. *J. Exp. Psychol. (Human Perception and Performance)* 6:590–604.

Moscovitch, M., Scullion, D., and Christie, D. (1976): Early vs. late stages of processing and their relation to functional hemispheric asymmetries in face recognition. *J. Exp. Psychol. (Human Perception and Performance)* 2:401–416.

Myers Pease, D., and Goodglass, H. (1978): The effects of cuing on picture naming in aphasia. *Cortex* 14:178–189.

Neilson, J. M. (1946): *Agnosia, Apraxia, Aphasia: Their Value in Cerebral Localization.* New York: Hoeber.

Neville, H. J. (1975): Cerebral specialization in normal and congenitally deaf children: An evoked potential and behavioral study. PhD dissertation. Cornell University.

Neville, H. J. (1977): Electrographic and behavioral cerebral specialization in normal and congenitally deaf children: A preliminary report. In: *Language Development and Neurological Theory.* Segalowitz, S., ed. New York: Academic Press.

Neville, H. J. (1980): Event-related potentials in neuropsychological studies of language. *Brain Lang.* 11:300–318.

Neville, H. J., and Bellugi, U. (1978): Patterns of cerebral specialization in congenitally deaf adults. In: *Understanding Language through Sign Language Research.* Siple, P., ed. New York: Academic Press, pp. 239–257.

Neville, H. J., and Hillyard, S. A. (1982): Neuropsychological approaches: State of the art report. In: *Animal Mind—Human Mind*. Griffin, D. R., ed. Heidelberg: Springer-Verlag, pp. 333–353.

Neville, H. J., Kutas, M., and Schmidt, A. (1982): Event-related potential studies of cerebral specialization during reading. II. Studies of congenitally deaf adults. *Brain Lang.* 16:316–337.

Newkirk, D. (1981): On the temporal segmentation of movement in American Sign Language. Manuscript. The Salk Institute for Biological Studies, La Jolla, CA.

Newkirk, D., Klima, E. S., Pedersen, C. C., and Bellugi, U. (1980): Linguistic evidence from slips of the hand. In: *Errors in Linguistic Performance*. Fromkin, V. A., ed. New York: Academic Press, pp. 165–197.

Newport, E. L. (1982): Constraints on structure: Evidence from American Sign Language and language learning. In: *Minnesota Symposium on Child Psychology* vol. 14. Collins, W. A., ed. Hillsdale, NJ: Lawrence Erlbaum.

Newport, E. L., and Ashbrook, E. (1977): The emergence of semantic relations in American Sign Language. *Papers and Reports on Child Language Development* 13:16–21.

Newport, E. L., and Supalla, T. (1980): The structuring of language: Clues from the acquisition of signed and spoken language. In: *Signed and Spoken Language: Biological Constraints on Linguistic Form*. Bellugi, U., and Studdert-Kennedy, M., eds. (Dahlem Konferenzen) Weinheim: Verlag Chemie, pp. 187–212.

North, E. (1971): Effects of stimulus redundancy on naming disorders in aphasia. PhD dissertation. Boston University.

Northup, L. R. (1977): Temporal patterning of grooming in three lines of mice: Some factors influencing control levels of a complex behaviour. *Behaviour* 61:1–25.

Ojemann, G. A. (1977): Asymmetric function of the thalamus in man. *Annals N.Y. Acad. Sci.* 299:380–396.

Ojemann, G. A. (1978): Organization of short-term verbal memory in language areas of human cortex: Evidence from electrical stimulation. *Brain Lang.* 5:331–340.

Ojemann, G. A. (1979): Individual variability in cortical localization of language. *J. Neurosurg.* 50:164–169.

Ojemann, G. A. (1980): Brain mechanisms for language: Observations during neurosurgery. In: *Epilepsy: A Window to Brain Mechanisms.* Lockard, J. S., and Ward, A. A., Jr., eds. New York: Raven Press, pp. 243–260.

Ojemann, G. A. (1981): Intrahemispheric localization of language and visuospatial functions: Evidence from stimulation mapping during craniotomies for epilepsy. In: *Advances in Epilepsiology, XII.* New York, Raven Press.

Ojemann, G. A., and Fried, I. (1982): Event related potential correlates of human language; cortex measured during cortical resections for epilepsy. In: *Advances in Epilepsiology: XIII Epilepsy International Symposium.* Akimoto, H., Kazamatsuri, H., Seino, M., and Ward, A., eds. New York: Raven Press, pp. 385–388.

Ojemann, G. A., and Mateer, C. (1979a): Human language cortex: Localization of memory, syntax, and sequential motor-phoneme identification systems. *Science* 205:1401–1403.

Ojemann, G. A., and Mateer, C. (1979b): Cortical and subcortical organization of human communication: Evidence from stimulation studies. In: *Neurobiology of Social Communication in Primates.* Steklis, H., and Raleigh, M., eds. New York: Academic Press, pp. 111–131.

Ojemann, G. A., and Whitaker, H. (1978): The bilingual brain. *Arch. Neurol.* 35:409–412.

Oller, D. K. (1980): The emergence of the sounds of speech in infancy. In: *Child Phonology*, vol. 1: *Production.* Yeni-Komshian, G. H., Kavanagh, J. F., and Ferguson, C. A., eds. New York: Academic Press, pp. 93–112.

Oppenheim, R. W. (1981): The neuroembryological study of behavior: Progress, problems and perspectives. In: *Models of Neural Development. Current Topics in Developmental Biology*, vol. 17. Hunt, R. K., ed. New York: Academic Press.

Oubredane, A. (1951): *L'Aphasie et l'Elaboration de la Pensée Explicite.* Paris: Presses Universitaires de Paris.

Padden, C. A. (1979): Verb classes in American Sign Language. Manuscript. The Salk Institute for Biological Studies, La Jolla, CA.

Padden, C. A. (1981): Some arguments for syntactic patterning in American Sign Language. *Sign Language Studies* 32:239–259.

Padden, C. A. (1982): Syntactic spatial mechanisms. Manuscript. The Salk Institute for Biological Studies, La Jolla, CA.

Padden, C. A., Bellugi, U., and Poizner, H. (1982): A case of Wernicke-like aphasia in a deaf man. Manuscript. The Salk Institute for Biological Studies, La Jolla, CA.

Paivio, A., and te Linde, J. (1982): Imagery, memory, and the brain. *Canadian Journal of Psychology* 36:243–272.

Patten, B. W. (1972): The ancient art of memory. *Arch. Neurol.* 26:25–31.

Pease, D. M., and Goodglass, H. (1978): The effects of cueing on picture naming in aphasia. *Cortex* 14:178–189.

Petersen, M. R., Beecher, M. D., Zoloth, S. R., Moody, D. B., and Stebbins, W. C. (1978): Neural lateralization of species-specific vocalizations by Japanese macaques (*Macaca fuscata*). *Science* 202:226–229.

Pick, A. (1913): *Die agrammatischen Sprachstorungen.* Berlin: Springer.

Poizner, H. (1981): Visual and "phonetic" coding of movement: Evidence from American Sign Language. *Science* 212:691–693.

Poizner, H., and Battison, R. M. (1980): Cerebral asymmetry for American Sign Language: Clinical and experimental evidence. In: *Recent Perspectives on American Sign Language.* Lane, H., and Grosjean, F., eds. Hillsdale, NJ: Lawrence Erlbaum, pp. 79–101.

Poizner, H., and Bellugi, U. (1980): Psycholinguistic studies of American Sign Language morphology. In: *Recent Developments in Language and Cognition.* Fokjaer-Jensen, B., ed. Copenhagen: University of Denmark, pp. 125–139.

Poizner, H., and Lane, H. (1979): Cerebral asymmetry in the perception of American Sign Language. *Brain Lang.* 7:210–226.

Poizner, H., Battison, R. M., and Lane, H. (1979): Cerebral asymmetry of American Sign Language: Effects of moving stimuli. *Brain Lang.* 7:351–362.

Poizner, H., Bellugi, U., and Lutes-Driscoll, V. (1981): Perception of American Sign Language in dynamic point-light displays. *J. Exp. Psychol. (Human Perception and Performance)* 7:1146–1159.

Poizner, H., Bellugi, U., and Tweney, R. (1981): Processing of formational, semantic, and iconic information in American Sign

Language. *J. Exp. Psychol. (Human Perception and Performance)* 7:1146–1159.

Poizner, H., Kaplan, E., Bellugi, U., and Padden, C. (1982): Cerebral specialization for nonlinguistic visual-spatial processing in deaf signers. Manuscript. The Salk Institute for Biological Studies, La Jolla, CA.

Poizner, H., Newkirk, D., Bellugi, U., and Klima, E. S. (1981): Representation of inflected signs from American Sign Language in short-term memory. *Memory & Cognition* 9:121–131.

Poizner, H., Herrera, M., Loomis, J. A., Bellugi, U., Livingston, R. B., and Hollerbach, R. (1981): Three-dimensional reconstruction and quantification of movement: Towards a visual-"phonetics" of a visual-gestural language. Manuscript. The Salk Institute for Biological Studies, La Jolla, CA.

Polit, A., and Bizzi, E. (1979): Characteristics of motor programs underlying arm movements in monkeys. *J. Neurophysiol.* 42:183–194.

Proudfoot, R. E. (1982): Hemispheric asymmetry for face recognition: Some effects of visual masking, hemiretinal stimulation, and learning task. *Neuropsychologia* 20: 129–144.

Pylyshyn, Z. W. (1977a): Children's internal descriptions. In: *Language Learning and Thought*. MacNamara, J., ed. New York: Academic Press, pp. 169–176.

Pylyshyn, Z. W. (1977b): What does it take to bootstrap a language? In: *Language Learning and Thought*. MacNamara, J. ed. New York: Academic Press, pp. 37–45.

Pylyshyn, Z. W. (1978): What has language to do with perception? Some speculations on the *Lingua mentis. American Journal of Computational Linguistics* 3:160–170.

Pylyshyn, Z. W. (1980): Computation and cognition: Issues in the foundation of cognitive science. *Behavioral and Brain Sciences* 3:111–132.

Pylyshyn, Z. W. (1981a): The imagery debate: Analogue media versus tacit knowledge. *Psychol. Rev.* 88:16–45.

Pylyshyn, Z. W. (1981b): Psychological explanation and knowledge-dependent processes. *Cognition* 10:267–274.

Pylyshyn, Z. W. (1982): *Computation and Cognition.* Cambridge, MA: Bradford/MIT Press.

Rand, T. C. (1974): Dichotic release from masking for speech. *J. Acoust. Soc. Amer.* 55:678–683.

Riedel, K. (1981): Auditory comprehension in aphasia. In: *Acquired Aphasia.* Sarno, M. T., ed. New York: Academic Press, pp. 215–270.

Riedel, K. (1982): Durational factors in the phonetic perception of aphasics. PhD dissertation. City University of New York.

Roberts, M., and Summerfield, Q. (1981): Audiovisual presentation demonstrates that selective adaptation in speech perception is purely auditory. *Percept. & Psychophys.* 30:309–319.

Roenker, A. L., Thompson, C. P., and Brown, S. C. (1971): Comparison of measures for the estimation of clustering in free recall. *Psych. Bull.* 76:45–48.

Roeper, T., and Siegel, M. (1978): A lexical transformation for verbal compounds. *Linguistic Inquiry* 9:199–260.

Rosenberg, B., Zurif, E. B., Garrett, M., and Bradley, D. (1982): Processing distinctions regarding open- and closed-class vocabulary items: New evidence from aphasia. Paper presented at: Academy of Aphasia, Mohunk, NY, October.

Ross, E. D. (1981): The aprosodias: Functional-anatomical organization of the affective components of language in the right hemisphere. *Arch. Neurol.* 38:96–101.

Ross, E. D., and Mesulam, M. M. (1979): Dominant language functions of the right hemisphere: Prosody and emotional gesturing. *Arch. Neurol.* 36:144–148.

Russel, W. R., and Espir, M. L. R. (1961): *Traumatic Aphasia: Its Syndromes, Psychopathology, and Treatment.* Oxford: Oxford University Press.

Safer, M., and Leventhal, H. (1977): Ear differences in evaluating emotional tones of voice and verbal content. *J. Exp. Psychol. (Human Perception and Performance)* 3:75–82.

Saffran, E. M., Schwartz, M., and Marin, O. (1980): The word order problem in agrammatism: II. Production. *Brain Lang.* 8:275–286.

Samuels, J. A., and Benson, D. F. (1979): Some aspects of language comprehension in anterior aphasia. *Brain Lang.* 10:263–280.

Schank, R. (1972): Conceptual dependency: A theory of natural language understanding. *Cognitive Psychology* 3:552–631.

Schlotterer, G. (1977): Changes in visual information processing with normal aging and progressive dementia of the Alzheimer type. PhD dissertation. University of Toronto.

Schlotterer, G., Moscovitch, M., and MacLachlan, D. (1982): Spatial frequency contrast sensitivity and visual masking in normal old people and patients with Alzheimer's disease. Manuscript.

Schwartz, M., Saffran, E. M., and Marin, O. (1980): The word order problem in agrammatism: I. Comprehension. *Brain Lang.* 10:249–262.

Searlman, A. (1977): A review of right hemisphere linguistic abilities. *Psychol. Bull.* 84:503–528.

Seashore, R. H., and Eckerson, L. D. (1940): The measurement of individual differences in general English vocabularies. *J. Educ. Psychol.* 31:14–38.

Semmes, J. (1968): Hemispheric specialization: A possible clue to mechanism. *Neuropsychologia* 6:11–26.

Sergent, J. (1982): The cerebral balance of power: Confrontation or cooperation. *J. Exp. Psychol. (Human Perception and Performance)* 8:253–272.

Sergent, J., and Bindra, D. (1981): Differential hemispheric processing of faces: Methodological considerations and reinterpretation. *Psychol. Bull.* 84:531–554.

Seyfarth, R. M., Cheney, D. L., and Marler, P. (1980): Monkey responses to three different alarm calls: Evidence of predator classification and semantic communication. *Science* 210:801–803.

Silverberg, R., Gordon, H. W., Pollack, S., and Bentin, S. (1980): Shift of visual field preference for Hebrew words in native speakers learning to read. *Brain Lang.* 11: 99–105.

Siple, P. (1978a): Constraints for sign language from visual perception data. *Sign Language Studies* 19:95–110.

Siple, P. ed. (1978b): *Understanding Language through Sign Language Research.* New York: Academic Press.

Smith, M. K. (1941): Measurement of the size of the general English vocabulary through the elementary grades and high school. *Genet. Psychol. Monogr.* 24:311–345.

Sperry, R. W. (1981): Changing priorities. *Ann. Rev. Neurosci.* 4:1–15.

Sperry, R. W., Gazzaniga, M. S., and Bogen, J. E. (1969): Inter-hemispheric relationships: The neocortical commissures; syndromes of hemispheric disconnection. In: *Handbook of Clinical Neurology*, vol. 4, chapter 14. Vinken, P. J., and Bruyn, G. W., eds. Amsterdam: North Holland, pp. 273–290.

Stark, R. E. (1980): Stages of speech development in the first year of life. In: *Child Phonology*, vol. 1: *Production*. Yeni-Komshian, G. H., Kavanagh, J. F., and Ferguson, C. A., eds. New York: Academic Press, pp. 73–92.

Stroop, J.-R. (1935): Studies of interference in serial verbal reactions. *J. Exp. Psych.* 18:643–662.

Stokoe, W. C., Casterline, D., and Croneberg, C. (1976): *A Dictionary of American Sign Language*. Silver Spring, MD: Linstok Press.

Studdert-Kennedy, M. (1976): Speech perception. In: *Contemporary Issues in Experimental Phonetics*. Lass, N. J., ed. New York: Academic Press, pp. 243–293.

Studdert-Kennedy, M. (1977): Universals in phonetic structure and their role in linguistic communications. In: *Recognition of Complex Acoustic Signals*. Bullock, T. H., ed. Berlin: Dahlem Konferenzen, pp. 37–48.

Studdert-Kennedy, M. (1980a): Language by hand and by eye: A review of Edward S. Klima and Ursula Bellugi's *The Signs of Language. Cognition* 8:93–108.

Studdert-Kennedy, M. (1980b): Speech perception. *Language and Speech* 23:45–66.

Studdert-Kennedy, M. (1981a): Cerebral hemispheres: Specialized for the analysis of what? *Behavioral and Brain Sciences* 4:76–77.

Studdert-Kennedy, M. (1981b): The beginnings of speech. In: *Behavioral Development*. Immelmann, K., Barlow, G., Petrinovich, L., and Main, M., eds. Cambridge: Cambridge University Press, pp. 533–561.

Studdert-Kennedy, M. (1982): On the dissociation of auditory and phonetic perception. In: *The Representation of Speech in the Peripheral Auditory System*. Carlson, R., and Granström, B., eds. New York: Elsevier Biomedical, pp. 9–26.

Studdert-Kennedy, M., and Lane, H. (1980): Clues from the differences between signed and spoken language. In: *Signed and Spoken*

Language: Biological Constraints on Linguistic Form. Bellugi, U.; and Studdert-Kennedy, M., eds. (Dahlem Konferenzen) Weinheim: Verlag Chemie, pp. 29–40.

Studdert-Kennedy, M., and Liberman, A. M. (1963): Psychological considerations in design of auditory displays for reading machines. *Proceedings of International Congress on Technology and Blindness* 1:289–303.

Studdert-Kennedy, M., and Shankweiler, D. P. (1970): Hemispheric specialization for speech perception. *J. Acoust. Soc. Am.* 48:579–594.

Summerfield, Q. (1979): Use of visual information for phonetic perception. *Phonetica* 36:314.

Supalla, T. (1982): Structure and acquisition of verbs of motion and location in American Sign Language. PhD dissertation. University of California at San Diego.

Supalla, T., and Newport, E. L. (1978): How many seats in a chair? The derivation of nouns and verbs in American Sign Language. In: *Understanding Language through Sign Language Research.* Siple, P., ed. New York: Academic Press, pp. 91–132.

Swinney, D. A. (1979): Lexical access during sentence comprehension: (Re) consideration of context effects. *J. Verb. Learn. Verb. Behav.* 18:645–659.

Swinney, D. A. (1982): The structure and time-course of information interaction during speech comprehension: Lexical segmentation, access, and interpretation. In: *Perspectives on Mental Representation.* Mehler, J., Walker, E. C. T., and Garrett, M., eds. Hillsdale, NJ: Lawrence Erlbaum, pp. 151–167.

Swinney, D. A., Zurif, E. B., and Cutler, A. (1980): Effects of sentential stress and word class upon comprehension in Broca's aphasics. *Brain Lang.* 10:132–144.

Tallal, P., and Newcombe, F. (1978): Impairment of auditory perception and language comprehension in dysphasis. *Brain Lang.* 5:13–24.

Thorne, J., Bradley, P., and Dewar, H. (1968): The syntactic analysis of English by machine. In: *Machine Intelligence,* vol. 3. Michie, D., ed. Edinburgh: Edinburgh University Press.

Timberlake, A. (1982): Invariance and the syntax of Russian aspect. In: *Tense and Aspect: Between Semantics and Pragmatics.* Hopper, P., ed. Amsterdam: John Benjamins B. V.

Tinbergen, N. (1951): *The Study of Instinct.* Oxford: Oxford University Press.

Tissot, R. J., Mounin, G., and Lhermitte, F. (1973): *L'Agrammatisme.* Brussels: Dessart.

Tomlinson, B. E., Blessed, G., and Roth, M. (1970): Observations on the brains of demented old people. *J. Neurol. Sci.* 4:205–242.

Trevarthen, C. (1979): Communication and cooperation in early infancy: A description of primary intersubjectivity. In: *Before Speech.* Bullowa, M., ed. Cambridge: Cambridge University Press, pp. 321–347.

Turvey, M. (1973): On peripheral and central processes in vision: Inferences from an information-processing analysis of masking with patterned stimuli. *Psychol. Rev.* 80:1–52.

Voegelin, C. F. (1935): *Tubatulabal grammar.* U.C.P.A.A.E. 34(2):55–190.

Von Stockert, T., and Bader, L. (1976): Some relations of grammar and lexicon in aphasia. *Cortex* 12:49–60.

Wapner, W., Hamby, S., and Gardner, H. (in press): The role of the right hemisphere in the apprehension of complex linguistic materials. *Brain Lang.*

Warden, C. J., and Warner, L. H. (1928): The sensory capacities and intelligence of dogs with a report on the ability of the noted dog "Fellow" to respond to verbal stimuli. *Quart. Rev. Biol.* 3:1–28.

Wasow, T. (1977): Transformations and the lexicon. In: *Formal Syntax.* Culicover, P., Wasow, T., and Akmajian, A., eds. New York: Academic Press.

Weigl-Crump, C., and Koenigsknecht, R. A. (1973): Tapping the lexical store of the adult aphasic: Analysis of the improvement made in word retrieval skills. *Cortex* 9:410–417.

Whitaker, H. (1979): Electrical localization and naming. Paper presented at: Conference on Neural Models of Language Processes, University of Massachusetts, Amherst, MA.

Wilbur, R. (1979): *American Sign Language and Sign Systems: Research and Applications.* Baltimore, MD: University Park Press.

Wilkins, A., and Moscovitch, M. (1978): Selective impairment of semantic memory after temporal lobectomy. *Neuropsychologia* 16:73–79.

Winner, E., and Gardner, H. (1977): The comprehension of metaphor in brain-damaged patients. *Brain* 100:717–729.

Woolridge, M. W. (1975): A quantitative analysis of short-term rhythmical behaviour in rodents. PhD dissertation. Oxford University.

Zaidel, D. W. (1981): Long-term memory and hemispheric specialization: Semantic organization for pictures. PhD Dissertation. Department of Psychology, University of California at Los Angeles.

Zaidel, D. W., and Sperry, R. W. (1977): Some long-term motor effects of cerebral commissurotomy in man. *Neuropsychologia* 15:193–204.

Zaidel, E. (1978a): Auditory language comprehension in the right hemisphere following cerebral commissurotomy and hemispherectomy: A comparison with child language and aphasia. In: *Language Acquisition and Language Breakdown: Parallels and Divergencies.* Carramazza, A., and Zurif, E. B., eds. Baltimore: The John Hopkins University Press, pp. 229–275.

Zaidel, E. (1978b): Concepts of cerebral dominance in the split brain. In: *Cerebral Correlates of Conscious Experience.* Buser, P. A., and Rougeul-Buser, A., eds. Amsterdam: North Holland, pp. 263–284.

Zaidel, E. (1978c): Lexical organization in the right hemisphere. In: *Cerebral Correlates of Conscious Experience.* Buser, P. A., and Rougeul-Buser, A., eds. Amsterdam: North Holland, pp. 177–197.

Zaidel, E. (1979): On measuring hemispheric specialization in man. In: *Advanced Technobiology.* Rybak, B., ed. Alphen aan den Rijn: Sijthoff and Noordhoff, pp. 365–404.

Zaidel, E. (1982a): Reading by the disconnected right hemisphere: An aphasiological perspective. In: *Dyslexia: Neuronal, Cognitive and Linguistic Aspects.* Zotterman, Y. ed. Oxford: Pergamon Press, pp. 67–91.

Zaidel, E. (1982b): Models of laterality effects in decoding words: A split-brain perspective. In: *Cerebral Hemisphere Asymmetry: Method, Theory and Application.* Hellige, J. B., ed. New York: Praeger.

Zaidel, E., and Peters, A. M. (1981): Phonological encoding and ideographic reading by the disconnected right hemisphere: Two case studies. *Brain Lang.* 14:205–234.

Zangwill, O. L. (1960): Speech. In: *Handbook of Physiology*, section 1, vol. 3: *Neurophysiology*. Field, J., Magoun, H. W., and Hill, K. E., eds. Washington, DC: American Physiological Society, pp. 1709–1722.

Zurif, E. B. (1974): Auditory lateralization: Prosodic and syntactic features. *Brain Lang.* 1:391–404.

Zurif, E. B. (1980): Language mechanisms: A neuropsychological perspective. *Am. Sci.* 68:305–311.

Zurif, E. B., and Blumstein, S. E. (1978): Language and the brain. In: *Linguistic Theory and Psychological Reality*. Halle, M., Bresnan, J., and Miller, G. A., eds. Cambridge, MA: MIT Press, pp. 229–245.

Zurif, E. B., and Caramazza, A. (1976): Psycholinguistic structures in aphasia: Studies in syntax and semantics. In: *Studies in Neurolinguistics*, vol. 1. Whitaker, H., and Whitaker, H. A., eds. New York: Academic Press, pp. 261–292.

Zurif, E. B., Caramazza, A., and Myerson, R. (1972): Grammatical judgments of agrammatic aphasics. *Neuropsychologia* 10:405–417.

Zurif, E. B., Caramazza, A., Myerson, R., and Galvin, J. (1974): Semantic feature representation in normal and aphasic language. *Brain Lang.* 1:167–187.